Air Fryer Cookbook 2021

2 books in 1: 100+ Amazing mouth-watering recipes to enjoy crispy dishes and wow your family. Lose weight fast and get lean in a few steps.

James Ball

Legal & Disclaimer

The information contained in this book and its contents is not designed to replace or take the place of any form of medical or professional advice; and is not meant to replace the need for independent medical, financial, legal or other professional advice or services, as may be required. The content and information in this book have been provided for educational and entertainment purposes only.

The content and information contained in this book have been compiled from sources deemed reliable, and it is accurate to the best of the Author's knowledge, information, and belief. However, the author cannot guarantee its accuracy and validity and cannot be held liable for any errors and/or omissions. Further, changes are periodically made to this book as and when needed. Where appropriate and/or necessary, you must consult a professional (including but not limited to your doctor, attorney, financial advisor or such other professional advisor) before using any of the suggested remedies, techniques, or information in this book.

Upon using the contents and information contained in this book, you agree to hold harmless the Author from and against any damages, costs, and expenses, including any legal fees potentially resulting from the application of any of the information provided by this book. This disclaimer applies to any loss, damages or injury caused by the use and application, whether directly or indirectly, of any advice or information presented, whether for breach of contract, tort, negligence, personal injury, criminal intent, or under any other cause of action.

You agree to accept all risks of using the information presented inside this book.

You agree that by continuing to read this book, where appropriate and/or necessary, you shall consult a professional (including but not limited to your doctor, attorney, or financial advisor or such other advisor as needed) before using any of the suggested remedies, techniques, or information in this book.

TABLE OF CONTENTS

INTRODUCTION **11**

THE AIR FRYER SECRETS............. **13**

Functions of Instant Pot.....................................15

Features and Specification 16

Safety features built within the Instant Pot.........................20

Control Panel 22

FAQ about the Duo Crisp Air Fryer.......................23

BREAKFAST RECIPES **25**

1. Breakfast Tarts.....................................25

2. Baked Eggs 27

3. Tomato Pepper Frittata 29

4. Tropical Oatmeal................................31

5. Simple & Easy Breakfast Casserole 32

6. Creamy Mac n Cheese 34

7. Cherry Risotto....................................36

8. Almond Coconut Risotto.....................38

9. Mushroom Frittata 40

10.   Morning Churros 42

LUNCH **44**

11.   Juicy Pork Chops 44

12.   Crispy Meatballs 46

13.   Flavorful Steak.. 48

14.   Lemon Garlic Lamb Chops 49

15.   Honey Mustard Pork Tenderloin 51

16.   Easy Rosemary Lamb Chops 53

17.   BBQ Pork Ribs 54

18.   Juicy Steak Bites 55

19.   Greek Lamb Chops 56

20.   Easy Beef Roast 57

DINNER **58**

21.   Thyme Turkey Breast.. 58

22.   Chicken Drumsticks 60

23.   Blackened Chicken Bake...................................... 62

24.   Crusted Chicken Drumsticks 64

25.   Brine-Soaked Turkey... 66

26.   Ground Chicken Meatballs 68

27. Easy Italian Meatballs 70

28. Oregano Chicken Breast 72

29. Lemon Chicken Breasts 74

30. Cajun Salmon 76

POULTRY **78**

31. Dry Rub Chicken Wings 78

32. Spicy Chicken Wings 80

33. Southwest Chicken Breasts 82

34. Simple Chicken Breast 84

35. Pesto Chicken Drumsticks 85

36. Herb Chicken Breast 87

37. Tasty Buffalo Chicken Wings 89

38. Asian Chicken Tenders 90

39. Curried Turkey Drumsticks 92

40. Dijon Drumsticks 94

FISH AND SEAFOOD RECIPES **97**

41. Spicy Prawns 97

42. Simple & Perfect Salmon 99

43. Healthy Salmon Chowder 100

44. Pesto Shrimp 102

45. White Fish with Cilantro Sauce 103

46. Sole with Mint and Ginger 105

47. Creamy Parmesan Shrimp 107

48. Delicious Garlic Butter Salmon....................108

49. Shrimp Mac n Cheese 110

50. Salmon Rice Pilaf...112

BREAKFAST RECIPES.................... 117

51. Creamy Polenta 117

52. Sweet Cherry Chocolate Oat.........................119

53. Farro Breakfast Risotto.................................121

54. Cajun Chicken 123

55. Tasty Chicken Tenders 124

56. Potato Fish Cakes 126

57. Baked Cod Fillet...128

58. Flavorful Chicken Skewers 130

59. Air-Fried Cinnamon & Sugar Doughnuts 132

60. Bok Choy And Spinach 135

LUNCH 137

61.   Herb Butter Rib-eye Steak..........................137

62.   Classic Beef Jerky....................................139

63.   BBQ Pork Chops......................................141

64.   Simple Beef Patties..................................143

65.   Simple Beef Sirloin Roast.........................145

66.   Seasoned Beef Roast.................................147

67.   Bacon Wrapped Filet Mignon....................149

68.   Beef Burgers...151

69.   Season and Salt-Cured Beef.......................153

70.   Sweet & Spicy Meatballs...........................155

DINNER **159**

71.   Buttered Salmon......................................159

72.   Lemony Salmon 161

73.   Miso Glazed Salmon 163

74.   Spiced Tilapia...165

75.   Crispy Tilapia...167

76.   Simple Haddock......................................169

77.   Crispy Haddock......................................171

78.   Vinegar Halibut.......................................173

79. Breaded Cod 175

80. Spicy Catfish 177

POULTRY 180

81. Delicious Fajita Chicken 180

82. Chinese Chicken Wings 182

83. Caribbean Chicken Thighs 184

84. Garlic Herb Chicken Breasts 186

85. Crispy Chicken Tenders.............................. 188

86. Cheese Herb Chicken Wings 190

87. Delicious Mustard Chicken Tenders 191

88. Baked Chicken Tenders 193

89. Paprika Chicken Breasts 195

90. Lemon Garlic Chicken Drumsticks 197

FISH AND SEAFOOD RECIPES 199

91. Perfect Salmon Dinner 199

92. Steam Clams 201

93. Delicious Tilapia.. 203

94. Horseradish Salmon 205

95. Shrimp Scampi 207

96. Dijon Fish Fillets..209

97. Garlic Parmesan Shrimp................................211

98. Bang Bang Breaded Shrimp 213

99. Taco Fried Shrimp...215

100. Asparagus Shrimp Risotto 217

CONCLUSION.................................. **220**

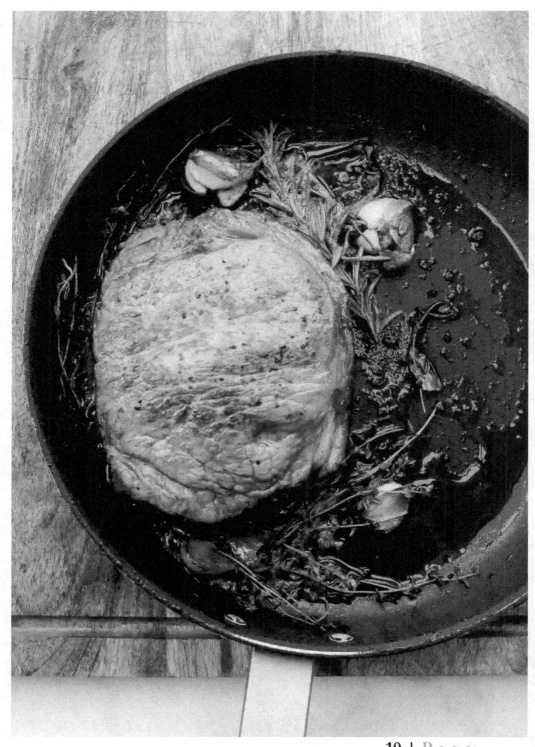

INTRODUCTION

The new air fryer is one of the multipurpose cooking appliances available now in the market. You will never need to buy another fryer that will help you lower your costs and save money. The lid of the Instant Fryer comes with Instant Clear Technology. It makes your food crispy on the outside and perforated on the inside, which also gives a nice brown texture to your food. The lid on the Instant Air Canister Fryer fries food in much less oil. If you are one of those people who likes fried food, but is also concerned about extra calories, then this kitchen appliance is for you. Makes your fries crisp on the outside and tender on the inside with a tablespoon of oil.

Instant Pot is not a new device for most people. Your food is delicious to seduce you and it shouldn't be unhealthy all the time. It's time for the new Instant Pot revolutions that are now being fried. This wonderful device combines science and art to bring you healthy meals for your whole family. Combining the dual functions of pressure cook and air fry, it allows you to prepare all kinds of pressure cook recipes as well as air fry recipes.

Instant Pot Air Fryer Crisp uses minimal cooking oil or fat, so you can enjoy a healthy air fry at home. Minimizes unhealthy fats, including trans fats and saturated, while keeping essential nutrients intact Instant Pot Air Fryer Crisp comes with many new options for steam, pressure, slow cooker, sous vide, roast, fries and chicken. Discover the secret to fast, healthy and delicious meals with this new kitchen appliance in this particular book. This book covers a detailed introduction to learn all about this new invention.

This is a complete book with a collection of recipes (Appetizers, Snacks, Poultry, Pork, Beef, Lamb, Fish, Seafood, Veggie, and Dessert) that you can cook effortlessly with the wonderful Instant Pot Air Fryer Crisp. Each recipe is tested to perfection and has been narrated with easy beginner instructions. Even if you are cooking for the first time, you can easily prepare all the recipes with simple instructions. Get ready for amazing food with crunchy, crunchy and caramelized foods. Let's find out what this new Instant Pot can do for you.

The Perks of Using the Duo Crisp Air Fryer. There are a lot of perks and benefits of using this appliance in your kitchen. Convenience, diversity, ease of use, tasty, and healthy food are only some benefits that scratch the surface. Let's know something more about how you can benefit from it.

The duality of functions facilitated by this device is something to be proud of. And looking at the control panel, you will get to know the broad scope of features that this device can perform with ease. I have been using two different appliances for pressure cooking and air frying. And let me tell you something that not even the individual appliances can perform these many functions as you are getting with this one.

Just swap the lid:

Turning your pressure cooker into an air fryer is only as hard as changing the lid. And if you would look at it, this changing of the lid transforms everything in your appliance. And to top that, you are well shielded from making any kind of mistake of mixing up the functions. Because you cannot operate the pressure cooker with the air fryer lid resting on the top of the appliance. And the same goes for when you are using it as a pressure cooker.

Placing the Lid:

The Air Fryer and Pressure cooker lid are easily locked in their place without obstructing the power cord outlet given on the appliance. The design is made to be simple and effective. And this is the case with every other Instant Pot appliance, they provide a safe and secure placement. Added to this, you will also get a separate tray to put the air fryer lid after use.

Easy to use Control Panel:

In other devices that have the same functionality or even the other Instant Pot appliances have preset functions. This literally confuses many users. But the Crisp Duo and Air Fryer do not have any such buttons to confuse you. It has just the primary function buttons provided on the front side of the pot. This time they have removed the buttons from the air fryer lid, too, and that is also something that I like about it.

Smart Accessories for a Smart Device:

Different accessories come as an add on with the Air Fryer Crisp Duo. For instance, the trivet that is made to place the food or even the pot after preparations are complete. Or, the double-layered air fryer basket is also something to be proud of with your appliance. Moreover, the multi-level air fryer basket, boiling or dehydrating tray, and the protective pad are some other essential accessories for this appliance.

One-Click Smart Functions:

Although there are no preset buttons on the appliance, you can work with some smart programs. For instance, the "Keep warm," or even the delay start button, adds another level of accessibility to the appliance.

Status Messages to your Rescue:

For a newbie, who is making their maiden attempt at cooking with the instant pot, there are status messages to help them understand their next steps. Messages like Lid, On, Off, Hot,

End, Food, and Burn indicate either the completion of a process or instruct you to take some action while cooking.

All the more, this book is best for those who are looking to start cooking for the first time with such a multi-tasking appliance. You will find information about what all you can do with this appliance along with how to use it best.

Functions of Instant Pot

The control panel of the Air fryer 11-in-1 Air Fryer/Electric Pressure Cooker is very easy to read and comprehend. Though the LED is small, the displays are easy to read, and interface navigation between the functions are relatively simple. Let us look at some quick highlights of the control panel that can help you understand the device better:

The time format on the control panel displays hours on the left and minutes on the right of the colon. Once the timer hits below 1 minute, the right side of the colon indicates the seconds remaining to complete the cooking.

Once the timer goes off, you will automatically see the light on the KEEP WARM button that will keep your food warm until you are back to check the cooker.

The control panel has no pre-sets; however, if you cook a specific dish multiple times, you can add it as a favorite pre-set to have the same function and settings every time you cook that meal.

On the control panel, you will see a button for DELAY START, which you can use if you want to cook a little later. It will ensure that the dish only cooks when you hit the START button, and until then, the panel will save your settings.

In case, if you want to cancel the meal preparation or wish to add or remove anything from the dish, you can always select the CANCEL button on the control panel, and the Instant Pot will immediately stop the cooking procedure.

The left side of the display is for the temperature setting. You can adjust the temperature by using the plus or the minus button.

On the right side of the display is for the timer. With the help of the plus and the minus button, you can change the timer setting.

The LED is a small black screen that appears on the control panel with blue scripts that signifies the settings you are using and also alerts if any of the devices/functions are missing in the Instant Pot.

Features and Specification

Functional Advantages and Applications:

Air Fryer: In this mode, you will have to use the crisp lid, instead of the pressure cooker lid. The function helps in frying the meals depending upon the temperature and time requirement. You can select the temperature after pressing on

AIR FRY,' and set/change the temperature and the time that you wish to cook and then press to START for beginning the cooking.

Default temperature: 400°F / 204°C

Temperature range: 180°F: 400°F / 82°C: 204°C

Suggested use: Fresh / Frozen fries, chicken wings or shrimps

Default cooking time: 00:18

Cooking time range: 00:01: 01:00

Roast: In this function, there is no pre-set, you can choose the temperature, and the time you require to roast your meal or dish and press START to begin the cooking process. Once you have maintained the temperature and the time, the Instant Pot will remember the pre-set in case if you wish to cook the same dish again.

Default temperature: 380°F / 193°C

Temperature range: 180°F: 400°F / 82°C: 204°C

Suggested use: Beef, Lamb, Pork, Poultry, Vegetables, Scalloped potatoes & more

Default cooking time: 00:40

Cooking time range: 00:01: 01:00

Bake: Using the air fryer lid, you can bake any dish that you want. The function remains the same, choose the temperature and the time and hit START to begin the baking process. Make sure to have the lid over the launching or cooling pad when you have finished the baking.

Default temperature: 365°F / 185°C

Temperature range: 180°F: 400°F / 82°C: 204°C

Suggested use: Fluffy and light cakes, pastries, and buns.

Default cooking time: 00:30

Cooking time range: 00:01: 01:00

Broil: In the BROIL option, the appliance comes with a 400°F default temperature setting, which you cannot change. Since it's a broiling option and it is the hottest setting, you can only change the time. Only after pressing the START option, the cooking will begin.

Default temperature: 400°F / 204°C

Temperature range: Not adjustable

Suggested use: Nachos, Onion Soup, Malt cheese, etc.

Default cooking time: 00:08

Cooking time range: 00:01: 00:40

De-hydrate: Just like any other pre-set, this one is also changeable, where you can change the temperature and timer as needed before you begin the process to DE-HYDRATE the meal.

Default temperature: 125°F / 52°C

Temperature range: 105°F: 165°F / 41°C: 74°C

Suggested use: Fruit leather, jerky, dried vegetables etc.

Default cooking time: 07:00

Cooking time range: 01:00: 72:00

Pressure cook: In this setting, it doesn't allow you to choose the temperature as the built-in option available are the frequencies of HIGH and LOW. By clicking on the pressure cook button, you can select the frequency, choose the time for the meal preparation, and hit START. Ensure to change the lid to the pressure cooker lid; otherwise, the control panel will refuse to begin the process.

Pressure level: LO (low: 8 to 2 psi) / HI (high: 12 to 16 psi)

Suggested use: LO: Fish and seafood, Soft vegetables, rice. HI: Eggs, meat, poultry, roots, hard vegetables, oats, beans, grains, bone broth, chili.

Default cooking time: LO: 00:35 / HI: 00:30

Cooking time range: 00:00: 04:00

Sauté: Under this function, it provides high or low-frequency operation and timer control. To begin the sauté, select the settings and press START.

Temperature level: LO (low) / HI (high)

Suggested use: LO: simmer, reduce, thicken, and caramelize. HI: pan sear, stir fry, sauté & brown.

Default cooking time: 00:30

Cooking time range: 00:01: 00:30

Slow Cook: The function is useful when you wish to slow cook the dishes. The timer of this function can go beyond 24 hours as per the recipe requirement, and the frequencies provided shall be either high or low as per the cooking requirements.

Temperature level: LO (low) / HI (high)

Suggested use: LO: All day cooking can set for 6 hours for the best results. HI: faster slow cooking.

Default cooking time: 06:00

Cooking time range: 00:30: 24:00

Steam: It is an ideal option when you wish to steam your dish like rice or dumplings, etc. The pre-set continues to remain the same with the frequency of high or low, and the timer can decide the steaming requirement.

Sous Vide: It is an ideal method for cooking the dish in the Instant Pot for non-fry cooking, which is especially useful for vacuum-sealed food cooking at a precise temperature for an extended period.

Default temperature: 56°C / 133°F

Default cooking time: 03:00

Cooking time range: 00:30: 99:30

Safety features built within the Instant Pot

When the pressure cooker is fully pressurized, you cannot open the lid until and unless the pressure is released. This feature has been incorporated to protect you from harm or damage due to an abrupt release of the lid forcefully.

Another good thing is that you cannot start cooking if the lid is not locked in its set place. Added to it, you will see a message "Lid" being displayed on the control panel.

There is a smart safety function that won't let the temperature go beyond a limit. These limitations are further set as per the program you have opted for preparing the dish.

The food items may get stuck at the bottom, or there is not enough liquid in the pot for the pressure cooker. In that case, there is overheating. To prevent any kind of damage, there is an overheating protection sequence that limits the formation of excessive heat.

The Instant Pot has an automatic pressure control system which maintains the pressure and suspends heating if the pressure inside the pot is more than the desired level.

There are features, specifications, and an introduction to the significant aspects of this book that you would want to know about. Other than this, you will get to read around 80 recipes that you can prepare with this appliance. Some of these recipes can be prepared with the pressure cooker and others with the air fryer. All of them are divided into different meal courses and kinds to help further you decide what you can eat for the morning breakfast, or evening snacks, or even for dinner.

Control Panel

The Instant Pot Crispy Air Fryer Lid is an attachment to the Air fryer Pressure Cooker. Simply put, the New Air fryer + Air Fryer combines air frying with the rest of cooking features with just a swapping of lids. While the pressure cooker lid offers the following functions:

Pressure cook

Sauté

Slow cook

Sous vide

Food warming

On the other hand, the Air fryer lid offers the following:

Air fry

Roast

Bake

Broil

Dehydrate

With its built-in smart programs, Instant Pot makes it easy for everyone to enjoy cooking whether they are chef or novice. Everyone can prepare their favorite healthy meal quick and fast.

FAQ about the Duo Crisp Air Fryer

What is the inner pot made of?

It is primarily made from 304 (18/8) stainless steel with the aluminum core at the 3-ply bottom for optimal use but ensures you that no aluminum comes in contact with the food you're cooking. There is also no aluminum coating and so the inner pot is in compliant with the FDA for safety standard requirements.

The steam rack is likewise made from food grade 304 (18/8) stainless steel, also ensuring safety for the food you're cooking.

The air fryer comes with a ceramic nonstick coating making food easy to remove and the air fryer basket easy to clean.

Can the setting be adjusted when you have started cooking?

Even when you have started cooking, you can still make some adjustments to the cooking time, cooking temperature, and pressure level.

How many appliances can the Air fryer + Air Fryer cover?

With the Air fryer + Instant Pot, you can have your traditional pressure cooker, steamer, slow cooker, food warmer, and sauté pan all in one kitchen device. Added to these, you can also make use of it as an air fryer, broiler, mini-oven, food dehydrator, and broiler.

Are there foods I should avoid putting into the Instant Pot?

Foods that are high in sugar content ay trigger the Instant Pot to give out a burn alert. Also, extra caution is highly recommended when cooking food like applesauce, oatmeal, pearl barley, and noodles that tend to froth, splatter, or foam as they can cause clogging. When preparing these types of foods, make sure not to fill it beyond the 1/2 line as indicated in the inner pot.

To ensure longevity, regular cleaning of the lids and all their parts are important for proper functioning.

Can I use accessories from other brands with my Air fryer + Air Fryer?

It is recommended that you purchase accessories and other spare parts only from stores authorized by Instant Pot Brands Inc. to ensure the highest level of safety.

1. Breakfast Tarts

Preparation time:10 minutes

Cooking Time: 12 minutes

Serving: 4

Ingredients:

- 1 sheet frozen puff pastry
- 4 tablespoons Cheddar cheese, shredded
- 4 tablespoons cooked ham, diced
- 4 eggs
- fresh chives, chopped

Directions:

1. Spread the pastry sheet on a flat surface and slice into 4 equal squares.
2. Place 2 pastry squares in the Air Fryer Basket.
3. Set the Air Fryer Basket in the Instant Pot Duo.
4. Put on the Air Fryer lid and seal it.
5. Hit the "Air fry Button" and select 6 minutes of cooking time, then press "Start."
6. Once the Instant Pot Duo beeps, remove its lid.

7. Press the center of each pastry square with the back of a spoon.
8. Add 1 tablespoon cheddar cheese, 1 tablespoon ham, and 1 egg to each of the square groove.
9. Return the basket to the Air fryer.
10. Put on the Air Fryer lid and seal it.
11. Hit the "Air fry Button" and select 6 minutes of cooking time, then press "Start."
12. Once the Instant Pot Duo beeps, remove its lid.
13. Cook the remaining pastry squares in a similar manner.
14. Garnish with chives.
15. Serve.

Nutrition: Calories 161 Total Fat 11.3g Saturated Fat 3.7g Cholesterol 176mg Sodium 241mg Total Carbohydrate 5.3g Dietary Fiber 0.3g Total Sugars 0.5g Protein 9.4g

2. Baked Eggs

Preparation Time: 10 minutes

Cooking Time: 8 minutes

Serving: 2

Ingredients:

- 2 eggs
- 1/4 cup spinach, chopped
- 1/4 onion, diced
- 1/4 tsp parsley
- 1/4 tsp garlic powder
- Pepper
- Salt

Directions:

1. Spray two ramekins with cooking spray.
2. In a small bowl, whisk together eggs, parsley, garlic powder, pepper, and salt.
3. Add onion and spinach and stir well.
4. Pour egg mixture into the prepared ramekins.
5. Place the dehydrating tray in a multi-level air fryer basket and place basket in the instant pot.
6. Place ramekins on dehydrating tray.

7. Seal pot with air fryer lid and select air fry mode then set the temperature to 350 F and timer for 8 minutes.

8. Serve and enjoy.

Nutrition: Calories 71 Fat 4.4 g Carbohydrates 2.1 g Sugar 1 g Protein 5.9 g Cholesterol 164 mg

3. Tomato Pepper Frittata

Preparation Time: 10 minutes

Cooking Time: 15 minutes

Serving: 2

Ingredients:

- 1 cup egg whites
- 1/4 cup tomato, sliced
- 1/4 cup pepper, sliced
- 2 tbsp milk
- Pepper
- Salt

Directions:

1. Add all ingredients into the large bowl and whisk until well combined.
2. Pour bowl mixture into the baking dish.
3. Place steam rack into the instant pot then place baking dish on top of the rack.
4. Seal pot with air fryer lid and select air fry mode and set the temperature to 320 F and timer for 15 minutes.
5. Serve and enjoy.

Nutrition: Calories 87 Fat 0.7 g Carbohydrates 5.6 g Sugar 2.2 g Protein 14.5 g Cholesterol 1 mg

4. Tropical Oatmeal

Preparation time: 10 minutes

Cooking time: 4 minutes

Servings: 4

Ingredients:

- 1 cup steel-cut oats
- 3 tbsp hemp seeds
- 1/2 papaya, chopped
- 1/2 cup coconut cream
- 2 cups of water

Directions:

1. Add oats, coconut cream, and water into the instant pot and stir well.
2. Seal pot with lid and cook on manual high pressure for 4 minutes.
3. Once done then allow to release pressure naturally for 10 minutes then release using the quick-release method. Open the lid.
4. Stir in hemp seeds and papaya.
5. Serve and enjoy.

Nutrition: Calories 195 Fat 11.2 g Carbohydrates 20.1 g Sugar 4.3 g Protein 5.5 g Cholesterol 0 mg

5. Simple & Easy Breakfast Casserole

Preparation time: 10 minutes

Cooking time: 20 minutes

Servings: 4

Ingredients:

- 2 1/2 cups egg whites
- 1/2 cup Mexican blend cheese
- 1/4 cup cream cheese
- 1/2 cup onion, chopped
- 1 cup bell pepper, chopped
- 1/2 tsp onion powder
- 1/4 tsp garlic powder
- 1/4 tsp pepper
- 1/4 tsp salt

Directions:

1. Spray instant pot from inside with cooking spray.
2. Add onion and bell pepper to the pot and cook until softened, about 5 minutes.
3. Transfer onion and bell pepper to the baking dish.
4. Add egg whites, seasonings, and cream cheese and stir well. Top with Mexican blend cheese.

5. Pour 1 cup of water into the instant pot then place the trivet in the pot.

6. Place baking dish on top of the trivet.

7. Seal pot with lid and cook on manual mode for 15 minutes.

8. Once done then release pressure using the quick-release method than open the lid.

9. Slice and serve.

Nutrition: Calories 208 Fat 10.4 g Carbohydrates 6.3 g Sugar 4.1 g Protein 21.7 g Cholesterol 33 mg

6. Creamy Mac n Cheese

Preparation time: 10 minutes

Cooking time: 5 minutes

Servings: 8

Ingredients:

- 15 oz elbow macaroni
- 1 cup milk
- 1/2 cup parmesan cheese, shredded
- 1 cup mozzarella cheese, shredded
- 2 cups cheddar cheese, shredded
- 1 tsp garlic powder
- 1 tsp hot pepper sauce
- 2 tbsp butter
- 4 cups vegetable broth
- 1/4 tsp pepper
- 1/2 tsp salt

Directions:

1. Add macaroni, garlic powder, hot sauce, butter, broth, pepper, and salt into the instant pot and stir well.
2. Seal pot with lid and cook on manual high pressure for 5 minutes.

3. Once done then release pressure using the quick-release method than open the lid.

4. Add cheese and milk and stir until cheese is melted.

5. Serve and enjoy.

Nutrition: Calories 388 Fat 15.3 g Carbohydrates 42.5 g Sugar 3.4 g Protein 19 g Cholesterol 43 mg

7. Cherry Risotto

Preparation time: 10 minutes

Cooking time: 10 minutes

Servings: 4

Ingredients:

- 1 1/2 cups arborio rice
- 1/2 cup dried cherries
- 3 cups of milk
- 1 cup apple juice
- 1/3 cup brown sugar
- 1 1/2 tsp cinnamon
- 2 apples, cored and diced
- 2 tbsp butter
- 1/4 tsp salt

Directions:

1. Add butter into the instant pot and set the pot on sauté mode.
2. Add rice and cook for 3-4 minutes.
3. Add brown sugar, spices, apples, milk, and apple juice and stir well.

4. Seal pot with lid and cook on manual high pressure for 6 minutes.

5. Once done then release pressure using the quick-release method than open the lid.

6. Stir in dried cherries and serve.

Nutrition: Calories 544 Fat 10.2 g Carbohydrates 103.2 g Sugar 37.6 g Protein 11.2 g Cholesterol 30 mg

8. Almond Coconut Risotto

Preparation time: 10 minutes

Cooking time: 5 minutes

Servings: 4

Ingredients:

- 1 cup arborio rice
- 1 cup of coconut milk
- 3 tbsp almonds, sliced and toasted
- 2 tbsp shredded coconut
- 2 cups almond milk
- 1/2 tsp vanilla
- 1/3 cup coconut sugar

Directions:

1. Add coconut and almond milk in instant pot and set the pot on sauté mode.
2. Once the milk begins to boil then add rice and stir well.
3. Seal pot with lid and cook on manual high pressure for 5 minutes.
4. Once done then allow to release pressure naturally then open the lid.

5. Add remaining ingredients and stir well.

6. Serve and enjoy.

Nutrition: Calories 425 Fat 20.6 g Carbohydrates 53.7 g Sugar 9.6 g Protein 6.8 g Cholesterol 0 mg

9. Mushroom Frittata

Preparation Time: 10 minutes

Cooking Time: 15 minutes

Serving: 2

Ingredients:

- 4 eggs
- 1 1/2 cups water
- 1/4 tsp garlic powder
- 4 oz mushrooms, sliced
- 1/8 tsp white pepper
- 1/8 tsp onion powder
- 2 tsp heavy cream
- 2 Swiss cheese slices, cut each slice into 4 pieces
- 1/4 tsp salt

Directions:

1. In a bowl, whisk eggs with spices and heavy cream.
2. Spray a 7-inch baking dish with cooking spray.
3. Add sliced mushrooms to the dish then pour egg mixture over the mushrooms.
4. Arrange cheese slices on top of the mushroom and egg mixture. Cover dish with foil.

5. Pour 1 1/2 cups of water to the instant pot then place steamer rack in the pot.

6. Place dish on top of the steamer rack.

7. Seal the pot with pressure cooking lid and cook on high for 15 minutes.

8. Once done, release pressure using a quick release. Remove lid.

9. Serve and enjoy.

Nutrition: Calories 264 Fat 18.5 g Carbohydrates 4.6 g Sugar 2.2 g Protein 20.6 g Cholesterol 360 mg

10. **Morning Churros**

Preparation time:10 minutes

Cooking Time: 5 minutes

Serving: 4

Ingredients:

- 1/4 cup butter
- 1/2 cup milk
- 1 pinch salt
- 1/2 cup all-purpose flour
- 2 eggs
- 1/4 cup white sugar
- 1/2 teaspoon ground cinnamon

Directions:

1. Melt butter in a 1-quart saucepan and add salt and milk.
2. Stir cook the butter mixture to a boil then stir in flour. Mix it quickly.
3. Remove the butter-flour mixture from the heat and allow the flour mixture to cool down.
4. Stir in egg and mix to get choux pastry and transfer the dough to a pastry bag.

5. Put a star tip on the pastry bag and pine the dough into straight strips in the Air Fryer Basket.

6. Set the Air Fryer Basket in the Instant Pot Duo.

7. Put on the Air Fryer lid and seal it.

8. Hit the "Air fry Button" and select 5 minutes of cooking time, then press "Start."

9. Once the Instant Pot Duo beeps, remove its lid.

10. Mix sugar with cinnamon in a mini bowl and drizzle over the churros.

11. Serve.

Nutrition: Calories 253 Total Fat 14.5g Saturated Fat 8.4g Cholesterol 115mg Sodium 166mg Total Carbohydrate 26.3g Dietary Fiber 0.6g Total Sugars 14.1g Protein 5.5g

11. Juicy Pork Chops

Basic Recipe

Preparation Time: 10 minutes

Cooking Time: 16 minutes

Servings: 4

Ingredients:

- 4 pork chops, boneless
- 2 tsp olive oil
- ½ tsp celery seed
- ½ tsp parsley
- ½ tsp granulated onion
- ½ tsp granulated garlic
- ¼ tsp sugar
- ½ tsp salt

Directions:

1. In a small bowl, mix together oil, celery seed, parsley, granulated onion, granulated garlic, sugar, and salt.
2. Rub seasoning mixture all over the pork chops.

3. Place pork chops on the air fryer oven pan and cook at 350 F for 8 minutes

4. Turn pork chops to other side and cook for 8 minutes more.

5. Serve and enjoy.

Nutrition: Calories 279 Fat 22.3 g Carbs 0.6 g Protein 18.1 g

12. Crispy Meatballs

Basic Recipe

Preparation Time: 10 minutes

Cooking Time: 12 minutes

Servings: 8

Ingredients:

- 1 lb. ground pork
- 1 lb. ground beef
- 1 tbsp Worcestershire sauce
- ½ cup feta cheese, crumbled
- ½ cup breadcrumbs
- 2 eggs, lightly beaten
- ¼ cup fresh parsley, chopped
- 1 tbsp garlic, minced
- 1 onion, chopped
- ¼ tsp pepper
- 1 tsp salt

Directions:

1. Add all ingredients into the mixing bowl and mix until well combined.
2. Spray air fryer oven tray pan with cooking spray.

3. Make small balls from meat mixture and arrange on a pan and air fry t 400 F for 10-12 minutes
4. Serve and enjoy.

Nutrition: Calories 263 Fat 9 g Carbs 7.5 g Protein 35.9 g

13. Flavorful Steak

Basic Recipe

Preparation Time: 10 minutes

Cooking Time: 18 minutes

Servings: 2

Ingredients:

- 2 steaks, rinsed and pat dry
- ½ tsp garlic powder
- 1 tsp olive oil
- Pepper
- Salt

Directions:

1. Rub steaks with olive oil and season with garlic powder, pepper, and salt.
2. Preheat the instant vortex air fryer oven to 400 F.
3. Place steaks on air fryer oven pan and air fry for 10-18 minutes turn halfway through.
4. Serve and enjoy.

Nutrition: Calories 361 Fat 10.9 g Carbs 0.5 g Protein 61.6 g

14. Lemon Garlic Lamb Chops

Basic Recipe

Preparation Time: 10 minutes

Cooking Time: 6 minutes

Servings: 6

Ingredients:

- 6 lamb loin chops
- 2 tbsp fresh lemon juice
- 1 ½ tbsp lemon zest
- 1 tbsp dried rosemary
- 1 tbsp olive oil
- 1 tbsp garlic, minced
- Pepper
- Salt

Directions:

1. Add lamb chops in a mixing bowl. Add remaining ingredients on top of lamb chops and coat well.
2. Arrange lamb chops on air fryer oven tray and air fry at 400 F for 3 minutes. Turn lamb chops to another side and air fry for 3 minutes more.
3. Serve and enjoy.

Nutrition: Calories 69 Fat 6 g Carbs 1.2 g Protein 3 g

15. Honey Mustard Pork Tenderloin

Basic Recipe

Preparation Time: 10 minutes

Cooking Time: 26 minutes

Servings: 4

Ingredients:

- 1 lb. pork tenderloin
- 1 tsp sriracha sauce
- 1 tbsp garlic, minced
- 2 tbsp soy sauce
- 1 ½ tbsp honey
- ¾ tbsp Dijon mustard
- 1 tbsp mustard

Directions:

1. Add sriracha sauce, garlic, soy sauce, honey, Dijon mustard, and mustard into the large zip-lock bag and mix well.

2. Add pork tenderloin into the bag. Seal bag and place in the refrigerator for overnight. Preheat the instant vortex air fryer oven to 380 Spray instant vortex air fryer tray with cooking spray then place marinated pork

tenderloin on a tray and air fry for 26 minutes Turn pork tenderloin after every 5 minutes. Slice and serve.

Nutrition: Calories 195 Fat 4.1 g Carbs 8 g Protein 30.5 g

16. Easy Rosemary Lamb Chops

Basic Recipe

Preparation Time: 10 minutes

Cooking Time: 6 minutes

Servings: 4

Ingredients:

- 4 lamb chops
- 2 tbsp dried rosemary
- ¼ cup fresh lemon juice
- Pepper
- Salt

Directions:

1. In a small bowl, mix together lemon juice, rosemary, pepper, and salt. Brush lemon juice rosemary mixture over lamb chops.
2. Place lamb chops on air fryer oven tray and air fry at 400 F for 3 minutes. Turn lamb chops to the other side and cook for 3 minutes more. Serve and enjoy.

Nutrition: Calories 267 Fat 21.7 g Carbs 1.4 g Protein 16.9 g

17. BBQ Pork Ribs

Basic Recipe

Preparation Time: 10 minutes

Cooking Time: 12 minutes

Servings: 6

Ingredients:

- 1 slab baby back pork ribs, cut into pieces
- ½ cup BBQ sauce
- ½ tsp paprika
- Salt

Directions:

1. Add pork ribs in a mixing bowl. Add BBQ sauce, paprika, and salt over pork ribs and coat well and set aside for 30 minutes
2. Preheat the instant vortex air fryer oven to 350 F. Arrange marinated pork ribs on instant vortex air fryer oven pan and cook for 10-12 minutes Turn halfway through.
3. Serve and enjoy.

Nutrition: Calories 145 Fat 7 g Carbs 10 g Protein 9 g

18. Juicy Steak Bites

Basic Recipe

Preparation Time: 10 minutes

Cooking Time: 9 minutes

Servings: 4

Ingredients:

1. 1 lb. sirloin steak, cut into bite-size pieces
2. 1 tbsp steak seasoning
3. 1 tbsp olive oil
4. Pepper
5. Salt

Directions:

1. Preheat the instant vortex air fryer oven to 390 F.
2. Add steak pieces into the large mixing bowl. Add steak seasoning, oil, pepper, and salt over steak pieces and toss until well coated.
3. Transfer steak pieces on instant vortex air fryer pan and air fry for 5 minutes
4. Turn steak pieces to the other side and cook for 4 minutes more.
5. Serve and enjoy.

Nutrition: Calories 241 Fat 10.6 g Carbs 0 g Protein 34.4 g

19. Greek Lamb Chops

Basic Recipe

Preparation Time: 10 minutes

Cooking Time: 10 minutes

Servings: 4

Ingredients:

- 2 lbs. lamb chops
- 2 tsp garlic, minced
- 1 ½ tsp dried oregano
- ¼ cup fresh lemon juice
- ¼ cup olive oil
- ½ tsp pepper
- 1 tsp salt

Directions:

1. Add lamb chops in a mixing bowl. Add remaining ingredients over the lamb chops and coat well.
2. Arrange lamb chops on the air fryer oven tray and cook at 400 F for 5 minutes
3. Turn lamb chops and cook for 5 minutes more.
4. Serve and enjoy.

Nutrition: Calories 538 Fat 29.4 g Carbs 1.3 g Protein 64 g

20. <u>Easy Beef Roast</u>

Basic Recipe

Preparation Time: 10 minutes

Cooking Time: 45 minutes

Servings: 6

Ingredients:

- 2 ½ lbs. beef roast
- 2 tbsp Italian seasoning

Directions:

1. Arrange roast on the rotisserie spite.
2. Rub roast with Italian seasoning then insert into the instant vortex air fryer oven.
3. Air fry at 350 F for 45 minutes or until the internal temperature of the roast reaches to 145 F.
4. Slice and serve.

Nutrition: Calories 365 Fat 13.2 g Carbs 0.5 g Protein 57.4 g

21. Thyme Turkey Breast

Preparation Time: 10 minutes

Cooking Time: 40 minutes

Serving: 4

Ingredients:

- 2 lb. turkey breast
- Salt, to taste
- Black pepper, to taste
- 4 tablespoon butter, melted
- 3 cloves garlic, minced
- 1 teaspoon thyme, chopped
- 1 teaspoon rosemary, chopped

Directions:

1. Mix butter with salt, black pepper, garlic, thyme, and rosemary in a bowl.
2. Rub this seasoning over the turkey breast liberally and place in the Air Fryer basket.
3. Turn the dial to select the "Air Fry" mode.

4. Hit the Time button and again use the dial to set the cooking time to 40 minutes

5. Now push the Temp button and rotate the dial to set the temperature at 375 degrees F.

6. Once preheated, place the Air fryer basket inside the oven

7. Slice and serve fresh.

Nutrition: Calories 334 Fat 4.7 g Carbs 54.1 g Protein 26.2 g

22. Chicken Drumsticks

Basic Recipe

Preparation Time: 10 minutes

Cooking Time: 20 minutes

Serving: 8

Ingredients:

- 8 chicken drumsticks
- 2 tablespoon olive oil
- 1 teaspoon salt
- 1 teaspoon pepper
- 1 teaspoon garlic powder
- 1 teaspoon paprika
- 1/2 teaspoon cumin

Directions:

1. Mix olive oil with salt, black pepper, garlic powder, paprika, and cumin in a bowl.
2. Rub this mixture liberally over all the drumsticks.
3. Place these drumsticks in the Air fryer basket.
4. Turn the dial to select the "Air Fry" mode.
5. Hit the Time button and again use the dial to set the cooking time to 20 minutes

6. Now push the Temp button and rotate the dial to set the temperature at 375 degrees F.

7. Once preheated, place the Air fryer basket inside the oven.

8. Flip the drumsticks when cooked halfway through.

9. Resume air frying for another rest of the 10 minutes

10. Serve warm.

Nutrition: Calories 212 Fat 11.8g Carbs 14.6 g Protein 17.3 g

23. Blackened Chicken Bake

Basic Recipe

Preparation Time: 10 minutes

Cooking Time: 18 minutes

Serving: 4

Ingredients:

- 4 chicken breasts
- 2 teaspoon olive oil
- Seasoning:
- 1 1/2 tablespoon brown sugar
- 1 teaspoon paprika
- 1 teaspoon dried oregano
- 1/4 teaspoon garlic powder
- 1/2 teaspoon salt and pepper
- Garnish:
- Chopped parsley

Directions:

1. Mix olive oil with brown sugar, paprika, oregano, garlic powder, salt, and black pepper in a bowl.
2. Place the chicken breasts in the baking tray of the Ninja Oven.

3. Pour and rub this mixture liberally over all the chicken breasts.

4. Turn the dial to select the "Bake" mode.

5. Hit the Time button and again use the dial to set the cooking time to 18 minutes

6. Now push the Temp button and rotate the dial to set the temperature at 425 degrees F.

7. Once preheated, place the baking tray inside the oven

8. Serve warm.

Nutrition: Calories 412 Fat 24.8 g Carbs 43.8g Protein 18.9 g

24. Crusted Chicken Drumsticks

Basic Recipe

Preparation Time: 10 minutes

Cooking Time: 10 minutes

Serving: 4

Ingredients:

- 1 lb. chicken drumsticks
- 1/2 cup buttermilk
- 1/2 cup panko breadcrumbs
- 1/2 cup flour
- 1/4 teaspoon baking powder

Spice Mixture:

- 1/2 teaspoon salt
- 1/2 teaspoon celery salt
- 1/4 teaspoon oregano
- 1/4 teaspoon cayenne
- 1 teaspoon paprika
- 1/4 teaspoon garlic powder
- 1/4 teaspoon dried thyme
- 1/2 teaspoon ground ginger
- 1/2 teaspoon white pepper

- 1/2 teaspoon black pepper
- 3 tablespoon butter melted

Directions:

1. Soak chicken in the buttermilk and cover to marinate overnight in the refrigerator. Mix spices with flour, breadcrumbs, and baking powder in a shallow tray.
2. Remove the chicken from the milk and coat them well with the flour spice mixture
3. Place the chicken drumsticks in the Air fryer basket of the Ninja Oven.
4. Pour the melted butter over the drumsticks
5. Turn the dial to select the "Air fry" mode. Hit the Time button and again use the dial to set the cooking time to 10 minutes
6. Now push the Temp button and rotate the dial to set the temperature at 425 degrees F.
7. Once preheated, place the baking tray inside the oven
8. Flip the drumsticks and resume cooking for another 10 minutes
9. Serve warm.

Nutrition: Calories 331 Fat 2.5 g Carbs 69 g Protein 28.7g

25. Brine-Soaked Turkey

Intermediate Recipe

Preparation Time: 10 minutes

Cooking Time: 45 minutes

Serving: 8

Ingredients:

- 7 lb. bone-in, skin-on turkey breast
- Brine:
- 1/2 cup salt
- 1 lemon
- 1/2 onion
- 3 cloves garlic, smashed
- 5 sprigs fresh thyme
- 3 bay leaves
- Black pepper
- Turkey Breast:
- 4 tablespoon butter, softened
- 1/2 teaspoon black pepper
- 1/2 teaspoon garlic powder
- 1/4 teaspoon dried thyme
- 1/4 teaspoon dried oregano

Directions:

1. Mix the turkey brine ingredients in a pot and soak the turkey in the brine overnight. Next day, remove the soaked turkey from the brine.

2. Whisk the butter, black pepper, garlic powder, oregano, and thyme. Brush the butter mixture over the turkey then place it in a baking tray.

3. Press "Power Button" of Air Fry Oven and turn the dial to select the "Air Roast" mode. Press the Time button and again turn the dial to set the cooking time to 45 minutes

4. Now push the Temp button and rotate the dial to set the temperature at 370 degrees F. Once preheated, place the turkey baking tray in the oven and close its lid.

5. Slice and serve warm.

Nutrition: Calories 397 Fat 15.4 g Carbs 58.5 g Protein 7.9 g

26. Ground Chicken Meatballs

Basic Recipe

Preparation Time: 10 minutes

Cooking Time: 10 minutes

Serving: 4

Ingredients:

- 1-lb. ground chicken
- 1/3 cup panko
- 1 teaspoon salt
- 2 teaspoons chives
- 1/2 teaspoon garlic powder
- 1 teaspoon thyme
- 1 egg

Directions:

1. Toss all the meatball ingredients in a bowl and mix well. Make small meatballs out this mixture and place them in the air fryer basket.

2. Press "Power Button" of Air Fry Oven and turn the dial to select the "Air Fry" mode. Press the Time button and again turn the dial to set the cooking time to 10 minutes

3. Now push the Temp button and rotate the dial to set the temperature at 350 degrees F. Once preheated, place the air fryer basket inside and close its lid. Serve warm.

Nutrition: Calories 453 Fat 2.4 g Carbs 18 g Protein 23.2 g

27. Easy Italian Meatballs

Basic Recipe

Preparation Time: 10 minutes

Cooking Time: 13 minutes

Serving: 4

Ingredients:

- 2-lb. lean ground turkey
- ¼ cup onion, minced
- 2 cloves garlic, minced
- 2 tablespoons parsley, chopped
- 2 eggs
- 1½ cup parmesan cheese, grated
- ½ teaspoon red pepper flakes
- ½ teaspoon Italian seasoning
- Salt and black pepper to taste

Directions:

1. Toss all the meatball ingredients in a bowl and mix well. Make small meatballs out this mixture and place them in the air fryer basket.

2. Press "Power Button" of Air Fry Oven and turn the dial to select the "Air Fry" mode. Press the Time

button and again turn the dial to set the cooking time to 13 minutes. Now push the Temp button and rotate the dial to set the temperature at 350 degrees F.

3. Once preheated, place the air fryer basket inside and close its lid.

4. Flip the meatballs when cooked halfway through.

5. Serve warm.

Nutrition: Calories 472 Fat 25.8 Carbs 1.7 g Protein 59.6 g

28. Oregano Chicken Breast

Basic Recipe

Preparation Time: 10 minutes

Cooking Time: 25 minutes

Serving: 6

Ingredients:

- 2 lbs. chicken breasts, minced
- 1 tablespoon avocado oil
- 1 teaspoon smoked paprika
- 1 teaspoon garlic powder
- 1 teaspoon oregano
- 1/2 teaspoon salt
- Black pepper, to taste

Directions:

1. Toss all the meatball ingredients in a bowl and mix well. Make small meatballs out this mixture and place them in the air fryer basket.

2. Press "Power Button" of Air Fry Oven and turn the dial to select the "Air Fry" mode. Press the Time button and again turn the dial to set the cooking time to 25 minutes

3. Now push the Temp button and rotate the dial to set the temperature at 375 degrees F.

4. Once preheated, place the air fryer basket inside and close its lid.

5. Serve warm.

Nutrition: Calories 352 Fat 14 g Carbs: 15.8 g Protein 26 g

29. Lemon Chicken Breasts

Basic Recipe

Preparation Time: 10 minutes

Cooking Time: 30 minutes

Serving: 4

Ingredients:

- 1/4 cup olive oil
- 3 tablespoons garlic, minced
- 1/3 cup dry white wine
- 1 tablespoon lemon zest, grated
- 2 tablespoons lemon juice
- 1 1/2 teaspoons dried oregano, crushed
- 1 teaspoon thyme leaves, minced
- Salt and black pepper
- 4 skin-on boneless chicken breasts
- 1 lemon, sliced

Directions:

1. Whisk everything in a baking pan to coat the chicken breasts well.
2. Place the lemon slices on top of the chicken breasts.

3. Spread the mustard mixture over the toasted bread slices.

4. Press "Power Button" of Air Fry Oven and turn the dial to select the "Bake" mode.

5. Press the Time button and again turn the dial to set the cooking time to 30 minutes

6. Now push the Temp button and rotate the dial to set the temperature at 370 degrees F.

7. Once preheated, place the baking pan inside and close its lid.

8. Serve warm.

Nutrition: Calories 388 Fat 8 g Carbs 8 g Protein 13 g

30. Cajun Salmon

Basic Recipe

Preparation Time: 5 minutes

Cooking Time: 10 minutes

Serving: 2

Ingredients:

- 2 Salmon steaks
- 2 tbsp Cajun seasoning

Directions:

1. Rub the salmon steaks with the Cajun seasoning evenly. Set aside for about 10 minutes. Arrange the salmon steaks onto the greased cooking tray.

2. Arrange the drip pan in the bottom of the Instant Vortex Air Fryer Oven cooking chamber. Select "Air Fry" and then adjust the temperature to 390 °F. Set the time for 8 minutes and press "Start".

3. When the display shows "Add Food" insert the cooking tray in the center position. When the display shows "Turn Food" turn the salmon steaks.

4. When the cooking time is complete, remove the tray from the Vortex Oven. Serve hot.

Nutrition: Calories 225 Carbs 0g Fat 10.5g Protein 22.1g

31. Dry Rub Chicken Wings

Preparation Time: 10 minutes

Cooking Time: 20 minutes

Servings: 4

Ingredients:

- 8 chicken wings
- 1/4 tsp black pepper
- 1/2 tsp chili powder
- 1/2 tsp garlic powder
- 1/4 tsp salt

Directions:

1. Line multi-level air fryer basket with parchment paper.
2. In a bowl, mix chili powder, garlic powder, pepper, and salt.
3. Add chicken wings to the bowl toss to coat.
4. Add chicken wings into the multi-level air fryer basket.
5. Place basket into the pot. Secure pot with air fryer lid and cook on air fry mode at 350 F for 20 minutes. Flip wings after 15 minutes.

6. Serve and enjoy.

Nutrition: Calories 557 Fat 21.7 g Carbohydrates 0.5 g Sugar 0.1 g Protein 84.6 g Cholesterol 260 mg

32. <u>Spicy Chicken Wings</u>

Preparation Time: 10 minutes

Cooking Time: 20 minutes

Servings: 3

Ingredients:

- 6 chicken wings
- 1 tbsp olive oil
- 1 tsp smoked paprika
- Pepper
- Salt

Directions:

1. Line multi-level air fryer basket with parchment paper.
2. In a bowl, mix chicken wings, paprika, olive oil, pepper, and salt.
3. Place marinated chicken wings into the refrigerator for 1 hour.
4. Add marinated chicken wings into the basket.
5. Place basket into the pot. Secure pot with air fryer lid and cook on air fry mode at 390 F for 20 minutes. Flip wings after 12 minutes.
6. Serve and enjoy.

Nutrition: Calories 640 Fat 27.3 g Carbohydrates 6 g Sugar 0 g Protein 85.5 g Cholesterol 260 mg

33. Southwest Chicken Breasts

Preparation Time: 10 minutes

Cooking Time: 25 minutes

Servings: 2

Ingredients:

- 1/2 lb. chicken breasts, skinless and boneless
- 1/4 tsp chili powder
- 1/2 tbsp olive oil
- 1 tbsp lime juice
- 1/8 tsp garlic powder
- 1/8 tsp onion powder
- 1/4 tsp cumin
- 1/8 tsp salt

Directions:

1. Line multi-level air fryer basket with parchment paper.
2. Add all ingredients into the zip-lock bag and shake well and place it in the refrigerator for 1 hour.
3. Add a marinated chicken wing into the basket.
4. Place basket into the pot. Secure pot with air fryer lid and cook on air fry mode at 400 F for 25 minutes. Turn halfway through.

5. Serve and enjoy.

Nutrition: Calories 254 Fat 12 g Carbohydrates 2.4 g Sugar 0.5 g Protein 33 g Cholesterol 101 mg

34. Simple Chicken Breast

Preparation Time: 10 minutes

Cooking Time: 12 minutes

Servings: 2

Ingredients:

- 2 chicken breast, skinless & boneless
- 2 tsp olive oil
- 1/2 tsp garlic powder
- Pepper
- Salt

Directions:

1. Line multi-level air fryer basket with parchment paper.
2. Brush chicken breast with oil and season with garlic powder, pepper, and salt.
3. Place chicken breast into the basket.
4. Place basket into the pot. Secure pot with air fryer lid and cook on air fry mode at 375 F for 12 minutes. Turn halfway through.
5. Serve and enjoy.

Nutrition: Calories 170 Fat 7.5 g Carbohydrates 0.5 g Sugar 0.2 g Protein 23.9 g Cholesterol 72 mg

35. Pesto Chicken Drumsticks

Preparation Time: 10 minutes

Cooking Time: 20 minutes

Servings: 4

Ingredients:

- 4 chicken drumsticks
- 1 tbsp ginger, sliced
- 8 garlic cloves
- 1/2 jalapeno pepper
- 1/2 cup cilantro
- 2 tbsp lemon juice
- 2 tbsp olive oil
- 1 tsp salt

Directions:

1. Line multi-level air fryer basket with parchment paper.
2. Add all the ingredients except chicken into the blender and blend until smooth.
3. Pour blended mixture into the mixing bowl.
4. Add chicken drumsticks into the bowl and stir well to coat.

5. Place marinated chicken drumsticks in the refrigerator for 2 hours.

6. Place marinated chicken drumsticks into the basket.

7. Place basket into the pot. Secure pot with air fryer lid and cook on air fry mode at 390 F for 20 minutes. Turn halfway through.

8. Serve and enjoy.

Nutrition: Calories 154 Fat 9.8 g Carbohydrates 3.3 g Sugar 0.4 g Protein 13.3 g Cholesterol 40 mg

36. Herb Chicken Breast

Preparation Time: 10 minutes

Cooking Time: 25 minutes

Servings: 2

Ingredients:

- 10 oz chicken breast halves
- 1/4 tsp dried thyme
- 1/4 tsp paprika
- 1 tbsp butter
- 1/4 tsp black pepper
- 1/4 tsp garlic powder
- 1/4 tsp dried rosemary
- 1/4 tsp salt

Directions:

1. Line multi-level air fryer basket with parchment paper.
2. In a small bowl, combine together butter, black pepper, garlic powder, rosemary, thyme, paprika, and salt.
3. Rub chicken halves with butter mixture and place into the basket.

4. Place basket into the pot. Secure pot with air fryer lid and cook on air fry mode at 375 F for 25 minutes. Turn halfway through.

5. Serve and enjoy.

Nutrition: Calories 324 Fat 16.3 g Carbohydrates 0.7 g Sugar 0.1 g Protein 41.2 g Cholesterol 141 mg

37. Tasty Buffalo Chicken Wings

Preparation Time: 10 minutes

Cooking Time: 24 minutes

Servings: 2

Ingredients:

- 1/2 lb. chicken wings
- 1/4 cup hot sauce

Directions:

1. Line multi-level air fryer basket with parchment paper.
2. Place chicken wings in the basket.
3. Place basket into the pot. Secure pot with air fryer lid and cook on air fry mode at 400 F for 24 minutes. Turn halfway through.
4. Transfer chicken wings to the bowl.
5. Add hot sauce and toss well.
6. Serve and enjoy.

Nutrition: Calories 219 Fat 8.5 g Carbohydrates 0.5 g Sugar 0.4 g Protein 33 g Cholesterol 101 mg

38. Asian Chicken Tenders

Preparation Time: 10 minutes

Cooking Time: 10 minutes

Servings: 3

Ingredients:

- 12 oz chicken tenders, skinless and boneless
- 1 tbsp ginger, grated
- 1/4 cup sesame oil
- 1/2 cup soy sauce
- 2 tbsp green onion, chopped
- 3 garlic cloves, chopped
- 2 tsp sesame seeds, toasted
- 1/4 tsp pepper

Directions:

1. Line multi-level air fryer basket with parchment paper.
2. In a large bowl, mix green onion, garlic, sesame seeds, ginger, sesame oil, soy sauce, and pepper.
3. Add chicken tenders into the bowl and coat well and place it in the refrigerator overnight.
4. Add marinated chicken tenders into the basket.

5. Place basket into the pot. Secure pot with air fryer lid and cook on air fry mode at 390 F for 10 minutes. Flip halfway through.

6. Serve and enjoy.

Nutrition: Calories 423 Fat 27.7 g Carbohydrates 6.4 g Sugar 0.9 g Protein 36.3 g Cholesterol 101 mg

39. Curried Turkey Drumsticks

Preparation Time: 10 minutes

Cooking Time: 22 minutes

Servings: 2

Ingredients:

- 2 turkey drumsticks
- 1/4 tsp cayenne pepper
- 2 tbsp red curry paste
- 1/4 tsp pepper
- 1/3 cup coconut milk
- 1 1/2 tbsp ginger, minced
- 1 tsp kosher salt

Directions:

1. Line multi-level air fryer basket with parchment paper.
2. Add all ingredients into the zip-lock bag, seal bag, and place in the refrigerator overnight.
3. Place marinated turkey drumsticks into the basket.
4. Place basket into the pot. Secure pot with air fryer lid and cook on air fry mode at 390 F for 22 minutes. Flip halfway through.
5. Serve and enjoy.

Nutrition: Calories 279 Fat 18.3 g Carbohydrates 8.4 g Sugar 1.5 g Protein 20.4 g Cholesterol 0 mg

40. Dijon Drumsticks

Preparation Time: 10 minutes

Cooking Time: 28 minutes

Servings: 2

Ingredients:

- 4 turkey drumsticks
- 1/2 tbsp ginger, minced
- 2 tbsp Dijon mustard
- 1/3 tsp paprika
- 1/3 cup sherry wine
- 1/3 cup coconut milk
- Pepper
- Salt

Directions:

1. Line multi-level air fryer basket with parchment paper.
2. Add all ingredients into the zip-lock bag, seal bag, and place in the refrigerator overnight.
3. Place marinated turkey drumsticks into the basket.
4. Place basket into the pot. Secure pot with air fryer lid and cook on air fry mode at 380 F for 28 minutes. Flip halfway through.

5. Serve and enjoy.

Nutrition: Calories 365 Fat 18.3 g Carbohydrates 5.3 g Sugar 1.9 g Protein 39.8 g Cholesterol 0 mg

41. Spicy Prawns

Preparation Time: 10 minutes

Cooking Time: 6 minutes

Serving: 4

Ingredients:

- 12 king prawns
- 1/4 tsp black pepper
- 1 tsp chili powder
- 1 tsp red chili flakes
- 1 tbsp vinegar
- 1 tbsp ketchup
- 3 tbsp mayonnaise
- 1/2 tsp sea salt

Directions:

1. Add prawns, chili flakes, chili powder, black pepper, and salt to the bowl and toss well.

2. Spray instant pot multi-level air fryer basket with cooking spray.

3. Add shrimp into the air fryer basket and place basket into the instant pot.

4. Seal pot with air fryer lid and select air fry mode then set the temperature to 350 F and timer for 6 minutes. Stir halfway through.

5. In a small bowl, mix together mayonnaise, ketchup, and vinegar.

6. Serve shrimp with mayo mixture.

Nutrition: Calories 254 Fat 5.9 g Carbohydrates 6.5 g Sugar 1.6 g Protein 43.2 g Cholesterol 636 mg

42. <u>Simple & Perfect Salmon</u>

Preparation Time: 10 minutes

Cooking Time: 7 minutes

Serving: 2

Ingredients:

- 2 salmon fillets, remove any bones
- 2 tsp olive oil
- 2 tsp paprika
- Pepper
- Salt

Directions:

1. Coat salmon with oil and season with paprika, pepper, and salt.
2. Place the dehydrating tray in a multi-level air fryer basket and place basket in the instant pot.
3. Place salmon fillets on dehydrating tray.
4. Seal pot with air fryer lid and select air fry mode then set the temperature to 390 F and timer for 7 minutes.
5. Serve and enjoy.

Nutrition: Calories 282 Fat 15.9 g Carbohydrates 1.2 g Sugar 0.2 g Protein 34.9 g Cholesterol 78 mg

43. **Healthy Salmon Chowder**

Preparation time: 10 minutes

Cooking time: 8 minutes

Servings: 4

Ingredients:

- 1 lb. frozen salmon
- 2 garlic cloves, minced
- 2 tbsp butter
- 2 celery stalks, chopped
- 1 onion, chopped
- 1 cup corn
- 1 medium potato, cubed
- 2 cups half and half
- 4 cups chicken broth

Directions:

1. Add butter into the instant pot and select sauté.
2. Add onion and garlic into the pot and sauté for 3-4 minutes.
3. Add remaining ingredients except for the half and a half and stir well.

4. Seal pot with lid and cook on manual high pressure for 5 minutes.

5. Once done then allow to release pressure naturally then open the lid.

6. Add half and half and stir well.

7. Serve and enjoy.

Nutrition: Calories 571 Fat 35.1 g Carbohydrates 26 g Sugar 3.9 g Protein 36.9 g Cholesterol 133 mg

44. Pesto Shrimp

Preparation Time: 10 minutes

Cooking Time: 5 minutes

Serving: 6

Ingredients:

- 1 lb. shrimp, defrosted
- 14 oz basil pesto

Directions:

1. Add shrimp and pesto into the mixing bowl and toss well.
2. Spray instant pot multi-level air fryer basket with cooking spray.
3. Add shrimp into the air fryer basket and place basket into the instant pot.
4. Seal pot with air fryer lid and select air fry mode then set the temperature to 400 F and timer for 5 minutes.
5. Serve and enjoy.

Nutrition: Calories 105 Fat 1.7 g Carbohydrates 2.9 g Sugar 0.2 g Protein 19.3 g

45. White Fish with Cilantro Sauce

Preparation time:10 minutes

Cooking Time: 30 minutes

Serving: 4

Ingredients:

- 1 large bunch of cilantros, chopped
- 1 small onion, chopped
- 3 cloves of fresh garlic, peeled and chopped
- 3 tablespoons butter
- 2 cups sour cream
- 2 teaspoons salt
- 4 tablespoons lime juice
- 2 1/2 pounds white fish fillets

Directions:

1. Add butter to a suitably sized skillet to melt over medium heat.
2. Stir in garlic and onion, then sauté for 5 minutes, then transfer to a blender.
3. Add cream, cilantro, salt, and lime juice, then puree this sauce until smooth.
4. Place the fish fillets in the Instant Pot Duo basket.

5. Put on the Air Fryer lid and seal it.

6. Hit the "Bake Button" and select 25 minutes of cooking time, then press "Start."

7. Once the Instant Pot Duo beeps, do a quick release and remove its lid.

8. Serve.

Nutrition: Calories 462 Total Fat 33.8g Saturated Fat 20.7g Cholesterol 135mg Sodium 1375mg Total Carbohydrate 11g Dietary Fiber 0.6g Total Sugars 1.7g Protein 29.9g

46. Sole with Mint and Ginger

Preparation time: 10 minutes

Cooking Time: 15 minutes

Serving: 4

Ingredients:

- 2 pounds sole fillets
- 1 bunch mint
- 1 2-inch piece ginger, peeled and chopped
- 1 tablespoon vegetable or canola oil
- 1/2 teaspoon salt
- 1/4 teaspoon freshly ground black pepper

Directions:

1. Add mint, salt, black pepper, ginger, and oil to a blender and blend until smooth.
2. Stir in 2 teaspoon water if the sauce is too thick then mix well.
3. Rub the fish with the mint sauce to coat it liberally.
4. Place the coated fish in the Instant Pot Duo.
5. Put on the Air Fryer lid and seal it.
6. Hit the "Air fry Button" and select 15 minutes of cooking time, then press "Start."

7. Once the Instant Pot Duo beeps, remove its lid.

8. Serve warm.

Nutrition: Calories 302 Total Fat 7.6g Saturated Fat 0.3g Cholesterol 147mg Sodium 559mg Total Carbohydrate 1g Dietary Fiber 0.3g Total Sugars 0g Protein 50.9g

47. Creamy Parmesan Shrimp

Preparation Time: 10 minutes

Cooking Time: 5 minutes

Serving: 4

Ingredients:

- 1 lb. shrimp, deveined and cleaned
- 1 oz parmesan cheese, grated
- 1 tbsp garlic, minced
- 1 tbsp lemon juice
- 1/4 cup salad dressing

Directions:

1. Spray instant pot multi-level air fryer basket with cooking spray.
2. Add shrimp into the air fryer basket and place basket into the instant pot.
3. Seal pot with air fryer lid and select air fry mode then set the temperature to 400 F and timer for 5 minutes.
4. Transfer shrimp into the mixing bowl. Add remaining ingredients over shrimp and stir for 1 minute.
5. Serve and enjoy.

Nutrition: Calories 219 Fat 8.4 g Carbohydrates 6.3 g Sugar 1 g Protein 28.4 g Cholesterol 248 mg

48. Delicious Garlic Butter Salmon

Preparation Time: 10 minutes

Cooking Time: 7 minutes

Serving: 4

Ingredients:

- 1 lb. salmon fillets
- 2 tbsp parsley, chopped
- 2 tbsp garlic, minced
- 1/4 cup parmesan cheese, grated
- 1/4 cup butter, melted
- Pepper
- Salt

Directions:

1. Season salmon with pepper and salt.
2. In a small bowl, mix together butter, cheese, garlic, and parsley and brush over salmon fillets.
3. Place the dehydrating tray in a multi-level air fryer basket and place basket in the instant pot.
4. Place salmon fillets on dehydrating tray.
5. Seal pot with air fryer lid and select air fry mode then set the temperature to 400 F and timer for 7 minutes.

6. Serve and enjoy.

Nutrition: Calories 277 Fat 19.8 g Carbohydrates 1.7 g Sugar 0.1 g Protein 24.3 g Cholesterol 85 mg

49. Shrimp Mac n Cheese

Preparation time: 10 minutes

Cooking time: 10 minutes

Servings: 2

Ingredients:

- 1 1/4 cups elbow macaroni
- 1 tbsp butter
- 2/3 cup milk
- 1 bell pepper, chopped
- 15 shrimp
- 1 tbsp Cajun spice
- 1/2 cup flour
- 1 cup cheddar cheese, shredded

Directions:

1. Add butter in instant pot and set the pot on sauté mode.
2. Add bell pepper and sauté for minutes.
3. Add water and pasta and stir well.
4. Seal pot with lid and cook on manual high pressure for 3 minutes.

5. Once done then release pressure using the quick-release method than open the lid.

6. Add Cajun spices and flour and stir well.

7. Set pot on sauté mode. Add shrimp and cook for 2 minutes.

8. Add cheese and milk and stir well.

9. Serve and enjoy.

Nutrition: Calories 843 Fat 30.2 g Carbohydrates 74.8 g Sugar 8.4 g Protein 65.1 g Cholesterol 429 mg

50. Salmon Rice Pilaf

Preparation time: 10 minutes

Cooking time: 5 minutes

Servings: 2

Ingredients:

- 2 salmon fillets
- 1 cup chicken stock
- 1 tbsp butter
- 1/2 cup of rice
- 1/4 cup vegetable soup mix
- 1/4 tsp sea salt

Directions:

1. Add all ingredients except fish fillets into the instant pot and stir well.
2. Place steamer rack on top of rice mixture.
3. Place fish fillets on top of rack and season with pepper and salt.
4. Seal pot with lid and cook on manual high pressure for 5 minutes.
5. Once done then release pressure using the quick-release method than open the lid.

6. Serve and enjoy.

Nutrition: Calories 474 Fat 17.4 g Carbohydrates 40 g Sugar 0.8 g Protein 39 g Cholesterol 94 mg

Air Fryer Cookbook for Beginners

The ultimate and most wanted cookbook for beginners, cook amazing dishes like a pro and wow your family

James Ball

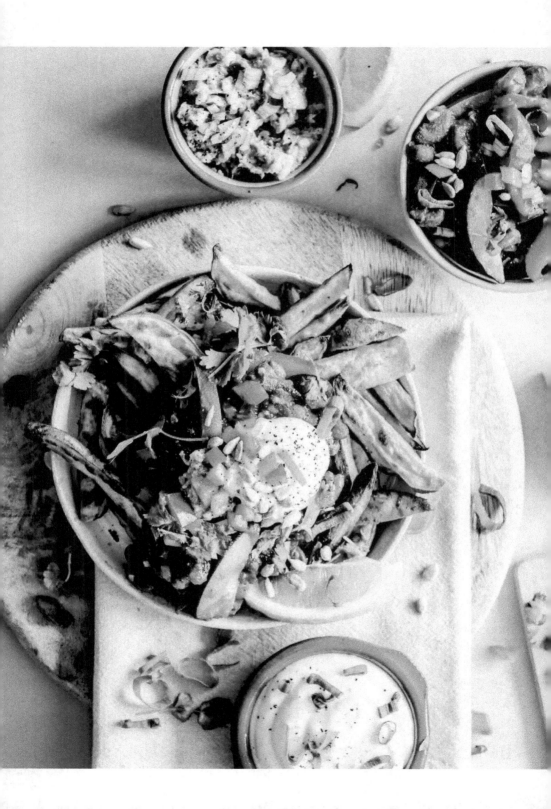

51. Creamy Polenta

Preparation time: 10 minutes

Cooking time: 5 minutes

Servings: 3

Ingredients:

- 1/2 cup polenta
- 1 cup of coconut milk
- 1 cup of water
- 1/2 tbsp butter
- 1/4 tsp salt

Directions:

1. Set instant pot on sauté mode.
2. Add milk, water, and salt in a pot and stir well.
3. Once milk mixture begins to boil then add polenta and stir to combine.
4. Seal pot with lid and cook on high pressure for 5 minutes.
5. Once done then allow to release pressure naturally then open the lid.

6. Stir and serve.

Nutrition: Calories 293 Fat 21.2 g Carbohydrates 24.7 g Sugar 2.9 g Protein 3.8 g Cholesterol 5 mg

52. Sweet Cherry Chocolate Oat

Preparation time: 10 minutes

Cooking time: 15 minutes

Servings: 4

Ingredients:

- 2 cups steel cuts oats
- 3 tbsp honey
- 2 cups of water
- 2 cups of milk
- 3 tbsp chocolate chips
- 1 1/2 cups cherries
- 1/4 tsp cinnamon
- Pinch of salt

Directions:

1. Spray instant pot from inside with cooking spray.
2. Add all ingredients into the pot and stir everything well.
3. Seal pot with lid and cook on high pressure for 15 minutes.
4. Once done then allow to release pressure naturally then open the lid.

5. Stir well and serve.

Nutrition: Calories 503 Fat 10.9 g Carbohydrates 85.5 g Sugar 22.5 g Protein 16.8 g Cholesterol 12 mg

53. Farro Breakfast Risotto

Preparation time: 10 minutes

Cooking time: 12 minutes

Servings: 4

Ingredients:

- 1 cup farro
- 1 tsp Italian seasoning
- 1/2 cup parmesan cheese, grated
- 1/2 cup mozzarella cheese, grated
- 2 tbsp heavy whipping cream
- 2 cups vegetable stock
- 1 tbsp butter

Directions:

1. Add butter into the instant pot and set the pot on sauté mode.
2. Add farro and cook for 2 minutes. Add stock and stir everything well.
3. Seal pot with lid and cook on manual high pressure for 10 minutes.

4. Once done then allow to release pressure naturally for 10 minutes then release using the quick-release method. Open the lid.

5. Add remaining ingredients and stir well.

6. Serve and enjoy.

Nutrition: Calories 206 Fat 13.7 g Carbohydrates 13.4 g Sugar 1.8 g Protein 9.9 g Cholesterol 37 mg

54. Cajun Chicken

Preparation Time: 10 minutes

Cooking Time: 15 minutes

Serving: 2

Ingredients:

- 2 chicken breasts, boneless & skinless
- 3 tbsp Cajun spice

Directions:

1. Season chicken breasts with Cajun spice from both the sides.
2. Place the dehydrating tray in a multi-level air fryer basket and place basket in the instant pot.
3. Place chicken breasts on dehydrating tray.
4. Seal pot with air fryer lid and select air fry mode then set the temperature to 350 F and timer for 15 minutes.
5. Serve and enjoy.

Nutrition: Calories 277 Fat 10.8 g Carbohydrates 0 g Sugar 0 g Protein 42.4 g Cholesterol 130 mg

55. Tasty Chicken Tenders

Preparation Time: 10 minutes

Cooking Time: 18 minutes

Serving: 4

Ingredients:

- 1 lb. chicken tenders
- 2 tbsp sesame oil
- 6 tbsp pineapple juice
- 2 tbsp soy sauce
- 1 tsp ginger, minced
- 4 garlic cloves, minced

Directions:

1. Add all ingredients except chicken in a bowl and mix well.
2. Add chicken and coat well. Cover and place in the refrigerator for 2 hours.
3. Place the dehydrating tray in a multi-level air fryer basket and place basket in the instant pot.
4. Place marinated chicken tenders on dehydrating tray.

5. Seal pot with air fryer lid and select air fry mode then set the temperature to 350 F and timer for 18 minutes. Turn chicken halfway through.

6. Serve and enjoy.

Nutrition: Calories 298 Fat 15.3 g Carbohydrates 4.9 g Sugar 2.5 g Protein 33.6 g Cholesterol 101 mg

56. Potato Fish Cakes

Preparation Time: 10 minutes

Cooking Time: 15 minutes

Serving: 4

Ingredients:

- 2 cups white fish
- 1 tsp coriander
- 1 tsp Worcestershire sauce
- 2 tsp chili powder
- 1 cup potatoes, mashed
- 1 tsp mix herbs
- 1 tsp mix spice
- 1 tsp milk
- 1 tsp butter
- 1 small onion, diced
- 1/4 cup breadcrumbs
- Pepper
- Salt

Directions:

1. Add all ingredients into the bowl and mix well to combine.

2. Make small patties from mixture and place in the refrigerator for 2 hours.

3. Place the dehydrating tray in a multi-level air fryer basket and place basket in the instant pot.

4. Place patties on dehydrating tray.

5. Seal pot with air fryer lid and select air fry mode then set the temperature to 400 F and timer for 15 minutes. Turn patties halfway through.

6. Serve and enjoy.

Nutrition: Calories 290 Fat 21.5 g Carbohydrates 13.8 g Sugar 2.1 g Protein 11.2 g Cholesterol 3 mg

57. Baked Cod Fillet

Preparation Time: 10 minutes

Cooking Time: 20 minutes

Serving: 4

Ingredients:

- 1 lbs. cod fillet
- 1 tbsp olive oil
- 1 tsp Italian seasoning
- 1/4 cup olives, sliced
- 1 cup cherry tomatoes, halved
- Pepper
- Salt

Directions:

1. Line instant pot multi-level air fryer basket with foil.
2. Coat fish fillet with oil and season with Italian seasoning, pepper, and salt.
3. Place fish fillet into the air fryer basket and place basket into the instant pot.
4. Add cherry tomatoes and olives on top of fish fillet.
5. Seal pot with air fryer lid and select air fry mode then set the temperature to 400 F and timer for 20 minutes.

6. Serve and enjoy.

Nutrition: Calories 143 Fat 5.9 g Carbohydrates 2.4 g Sugar 1.3 g Protein 20.7 g Cholesterol 57 mg

58. Flavorful Chicken Skewers

Preparation Time: 10 minutes

Cooking Time: 20 minutes

Serving: 4

Ingredients:

- 1 1/2 lbs. chicken breast, cut into 1-inch cubes
- For marinade:
- 1/4 cup fresh mint leaves
- 5 garlic cloves
- 1/2 cup lemon juice
- 1/4 tsp cayenne
- 1 cup olive oil
- 1 tbsp vinegar
- 1/2 cup yogurt
- 2 tbsp fresh rosemary, chopped
- 2 tbsp dried oregano
- Pepper
- Salt

Directions:

1. Add all marinade ingredients into the blender and blend until smooth.

2. Pour marinade in a mixing bowl.

3. Add chicken to the bowl and coat well and place it in the refrigerator for 1 hour.

4. Thread marinated chicken onto the soaked wooden skewers.

5. Spray instant pot multi-level air fryer basket with cooking spray.

6. Place chicken skewers into the air fryer basket and place basket into the instant pot.

7. Seal pot with air fryer lid and select air fry mode then set the temperature to 400 F and timer for 20 minutes. Turn halfway through.

8. Serve and enjoy.

Nutrition: Calories 677 Fat 55.8 g Carbohydrates 7.1 g Sugar 3 g Protein 38.8 g Cholesterol 111 mg

59. Air-Fried Cinnamon & Sugar Doughnuts

Preparation: 25 minutes

Cooking: 8 minutes

Servings: 9

Ingredients:

- 2¼ + ¼ cup all-purpose flour
- ¾ + 1/3 cup white sugar
- 2 egg yolks, large
- 2½ tablespoons butter kept in room temperature
- 1½ teaspoons baking powder
- ½ cup sour cream
- 2 tablespoons butter, melted
- 1 teaspoon cinnamon
- 1 teaspoon salt

Directions:

1. In a bowl combine, 2½ tablespoon butter kept in room temperature with ¾ cup white sugar, until it takes a crumbly shape.

2. Now add the egg yolk and mix thoroughly.

3. Put the all-purpose flour, salt, and baking powder in a medium bowl and combine.

4. Put one-third of the flour mixture into the egg-sugar mix and combine thoroughly.

5. Add the remaining flour and sour cream and mix well.

6. Refrigerate the mixture for 3-4 hours.

7. Mix cinnamon and 1/3 cup of white sugar in another medium bowl.

8. Keep ready your kitchen working table and spread some flour on it.

9. Take out the refrigerated dough and spread it into ½" thick sheet.

10. Cut it into 9 large dough using a dough dye cutter and make a small circle in the center of each dough, to make it look like a dough.

11. Place the air fryer basket in the inner pot of the Instant Pot Air Fryer.

12. Close the crisp cover of your Instant Pot Air Fryer and preheat at 340°F for 3 minutes in the AIR FRYER mode.

13. Press START to begin preheating.

14. Apply melted butter on both sides of the doughnut before placing it in the air fryer.

15. Place the doughs in the basket without overlapping.

16. If space is not enough, use the separator and place the remaining dough on it.

17. Close the crisp lid.

18. Set the timer to 8 minutes and temperature at 340°F.

19. Press START for cooking.

20. Brush the melted butter on the cooked doughnuts and dredge it into the cinnamon-sugar mixture.

21. Your doughnuts are ready to serve.

Nutrition: Calories: 276, Total fat: 9.7g, Saturated fat: 6g, Cholesterol: 66mg, Sodium: 390mg, Protein: 4.3g, Potassium: 59mg, Total carbs: 43.5g, Dietary fiber: 1g, Sugars: 19g.

60. Bok Choy And Spinach

Preparation time: 20 minutes

Cooking Time: 30 minutes

Servings: 4

Ingredients:

- 3 oz. Mozzarella; shredded
- 7oz. Baby spinach; torn
- 7 oz. Bok choy; torn
- 2 eggs; whisked
- 2 tbsp. Olive oil
- 2 tbsp. Coconut cream
- Salt and black pepper to taste.

Directions:

1. In your air fryer, combine all the ingredients except the mozzarella and toss them gently.
2. Sprinkle the mozzarella on top, cook at 360°f for 15 minutes.
3. Divide between plates and serve

Nutrition: Calories: 200; Fat: 12g; Fiber: 2g; Carbs: 3g; Protein: 8g

61. Herb Butter Rib-eye Steak

Basic Recipe

Preparation Time: 10 minutes

Cooking Time: 14 minutes

Servings: 4

Ingredients:

- 2 lbs. rib eye steak, bone-in
- 1 tsp fresh rosemary, chopped
- 1 tsp fresh thyme, chopped
- 1 tsp fresh chives, chopped
- 2 tsp fresh parsley, chopped
- 1 tsp garlic, minced
- ¼ cup butter softened
- Pepper
- Salt

Directions:

1. In a small bowl, combine together butter and herbs.
2. Rub herb butter on rib-eye steak and place it in the refrigerator for 30 minutes

3. Place marinated steak on instant vortex air fryer oven pan and cook at 400 F for 12-14 minutes
4. Serve and enjoy.

Nutrition: Calories 416 Fat 36.7 g Carbs 0.7 g Protein 20.3 g

62. Classic Beef Jerky

Basic Recipe

Preparation Time: 10 minutes

Cooking Time: 4 hours

Servings: 4

Ingredients:

- 2 lbs. London broil, sliced thinly
- 1 tsp onion powder
- 3 tbsp brown sugar
- 3 tbsp soy sauce
- 1 tsp olive oil
- 3/4 tsp garlic powder

Directions:

1. Add all ingredients except meat in the large zip-lock bag.
2. Mix until well combined. Add meat in the bag.
3. Seal bag and massage gently to cover the meat with marinade.
4. Let marinate the meat for 1 hour.
5. Arrange marinated meat slices on instant vortex air fryer tray and dehydrate at 160 F for 4 hours.

Nutrition: Calories 133 Fat 4.7 g Carbs 9.4 g Protein 13.4 g

63. BBQ Pork Chops

Basic Recipe

Preparation Time: 10 minutes

Cooking Time: 7 minutes

Servings: 4

Ingredients:

- 4 pork chops
- For rub:
- ½ tsp allspice
- ½ tsp dry mustard
- 1 tsp ground cumin
- 1 tsp garlic powder
- ½ tsp chili powder
- ½ tsp paprika
- 1 tbsp brown sugar
- 1 tsp salt

Directions:

1. In a small bowl, mix together all rub ingredients and rub all over pork chops.
2. Arrange pork chops on air fryer tray and air fry at 400 F for 5.

3. Turn pork chops to other side and air fry for 2 minutes more.

4. Serve and enjoy.

Nutrition: Calories 273 Fat 20.2 g Carbs 3.4 g Protein 18.4 g

64. Simple Beef Patties

Basic Recipe

Preparation Time: 10 minutes

Cooking Time: 13 minutes

Servings: 4

Ingredients:

- 1 lb. ground beef
- ½ tsp garlic powder
- ¼ tsp onion powder
- Pepper
- Salt

Directions:

1. Preheat the instant vortex air fryer oven to 400 F.
2. Add ground meat, garlic powder, onion powder, pepper, and salt into the mixing bowl and mix until well combined.
3. Make even shape patties from meat mixture and arrange on air fryer pan.
4. Place pan in instant vortex air fryer oven.
5. Cook patties for 10 minutes Turn patties after 5 minutes
6. Serve and enjoy.

Nutrition: Calories 212 Fat 7.1 g Carbs 0.4 g Protein 34.5 g

65. Simple Beef Sirloin Roast

Basic Recipe
Preparation Time: 10 minutes
Cooking Time: 50 minutes
Servings: 8

Ingredients:

- 2½ pounds sirloin roast
- Salt and ground black pepper, as required

Directions:

1. Rub the roast with salt and black pepper generously.
2. Insert the rotisserie rod through the roast.
3. Insert the rotisserie forks, one on each side of the rod to secure the rod to the chicken.
4. Arrange the drip pan in the bottom of Instant Vortex Plus Air Fryer Oven cooking chamber.
5. Select "Roast" and then adjust the temperature to 350 degrees F.
6. Set the timer for 50 minutes and press the "Start".
7. When the display shows "Add Food" press the red lever down and load the left side of the rod into the Vortex.

8. Now, slide the rod's left side into the groove along the metal bar so it doesn't move. Then, close the door and touch "Rotate". Press the red lever to release the rod when cooking time is complete.

9. Remove from the Vortex and place the roast onto a platter for about 10 minutes before slicing. With a sharp knife, cut the roast into desired sized slices and serve.

Nutrition: Calories 201 Fat 8.8 g Carbs 0 g Protein 28.9 g

66. Seasoned Beef Roast

Basic Recipe

Preparation Time: 10 minutes

Cooking Time: 45 minutes

Servings: 10

Ingredients:

- 3 pounds beef top roast
- 1 tablespoon olive oil
- 2 tablespoons Montreal steak seasoning

Directions:

1. Coat the roast with oil and then rub with the seasoning generously.
2. With kitchen twines, tie the roast to keep it compact. Arrange the roast onto the cooking tray.
3. Arrange the drip pan in the bottom of Instant Vortex plus Air Fryer Oven cooking chamber.
4. Select "Air Fry" and then adjust the temperature to 360 degrees F. Set the timer for 45 minutes and press the "Start".
5. When the display shows "Add Food" insert the cooking tray in the center position.
6. When the display shows "Turn Food" do nothing.

7. When cooking time is complete, remove the tray from Vortex and place the roast onto a platter for about 10 minutes before slicing. With a sharp knife, cut the roast into desired sized slices and serve.

Nutrition: Calories 269 Fat 9.9 g Carbs 0 g Fiber 0 g

67. Bacon Wrapped Filet Mignon

Basic Recipe

Preparation Time: 10 minutes

Cooking Time: 15 minutes

Servings: 2

Ingredients:

- 2 bacon slices
- 2 (4-ounce) filet mignon
- Salt and ground black pepper, as required
- Olive oil cooking spray

Directions:

1. Wrap 1 bacon slice around each filet mignon and secure with toothpicks.
2. Season the filets with the salt and black pepper lightly.
3. Arrange the filet mignon onto a coking rack and spray with cooking spray.
4. Arrange the drip pan in the bottom of Instant Vortex plus Air Fryer Oven cooking chamber.
5. Select "Air Fry" and then adjust the temperature to 375 degrees F.
6. Set the timer for 15 minutes and press the "Start".

7. When the display shows "Add Food" insert the cooking rack in the center position.

8. When the display shows "Turn Food" turn the filets.

9. When cooking time is complete, remove the rack from Vortex and serve hot.

Nutrition: Calories 360 Fat 19.6 g Carbs 0.4 g Protein 42.6 g

68. Beef Burgers

Basic Recipe

Preparation Time: 15 minutes

Cooking Time: 18 minutes

Servings: 4

Ingredients:

- For Burgers:
- 1-pound ground beef
- ½ cup panko breadcrumbs
- ¼ cup onion, chopped finely
- 3 tablespoons Dijon mustard
- 3 teaspoons low-sodium soy sauce
- 2 teaspoons fresh rosemary, chopped finely
- Salt, to taste
- For Topping:
- 2 tablespoons Dijon mustard
- 1 tablespoon brown sugar
- 1 teaspoon soy sauce
- 4 Gruyere cheese slices

Directions:

1. In a large bowl, add all the ingredients and mix until well combined.
2. Make 4 equal-sized patties from the mixture.
3. Arrange the patties onto a cooking tray.
4. Arrange the drip pan in the bottom of Instant Vortex Plus Air Fryer Oven cooking chamber.
5. Select "Air Fry" and then adjust the temperature to 370 degrees F.
6. Set the timer for 15 minutes and press the "Start".
7. When the display shows "Add Food" insert the cooking rack in the center position.
8. When the display shows "Turn Food" turn the burgers.
9. Meanwhile, for sauce: in a small bowl, add the mustard, brown sugar and soy sauce and mix well.
10. When cooking time is complete, remove the tray from Vortex and coat the burgers with the sauce.
11. Top each burger with 1 cheese slice.
12. Return the tray to the cooking chamber and select "Broil".
13. Set the timer for 3 minutes and press the "Start".
14. When cooking time is complete, remove the tray from Vortex and serve hot.

Nutrition: Calories 402 Fat 18 g Carbs 6.3 g Protein 44.4 g

69. Season and Salt-Cured Beef

Intermediate Recipe

Preparation Time: 15 minutes

Cooking Time: 3 hours

Servings: 4

Ingredients:

- 1½ pounds beef round, trimmed
- ½ cup Worcestershire sauce
- ½ cup low-sodium soy sauce
- 2 teaspoons honey
- 1 teaspoon liquid smoke
- 2 teaspoons onion powder
- ½ teaspoon red pepper flakes
- Ground black pepper, as required

Directions:

1. In a zip-top bag, place the beef and freeze for 1-2 hours to firm up.
2. Place the meat onto a cutting board and cut against the grain into 1/8-¼-inch strips.
3. In a large bowl, add the remaining ingredients and mix until well combined.

4. Add the steak slices and coat with the mixture generously.

5. Refrigerate to marinate for about 4-6 hours.

6. Remove the beef slices from bowl and with paper towels, pat dry them.

7. Divide the steak strips onto the cooking trays and arrange in an even layer.

8. Select "Dehydrate" and then adjust the temperature to 160 degrees F.

9. Set the timer for 3 hours and press the "Start".

10. When the display shows "Add Food" insert 1 tray in the top position and another in the center position.

11. After 1½ hours, switch the position of cooking trays.

12. Meanwhile, in a small pan, add the remaining ingredients over medium heat and cook for about 10 minutes, stirring occasionally.

13. When cooking time is complete, remove the trays from Vortex.

Nutrition: Calories 372 Fat 10.7 g Carbs 12 g Protein 53.8 g

70. Sweet & Spicy Meatballs

Basic Recipe

Preparation Time: 20 minutes

Cooking Time: 30 minutes

Servings: 8

Ingredients:

For Meatballs:

- 2 pounds lean ground beef
- 2/3 cup quick-cooking oats
- ½ cup Ritz crackers, crushed
- 1 (5-ounce) can evaporated milk
- 2 large eggs, beaten lightly
- 1 teaspoon honey
- 1 tablespoon dried onion, minced
- 1 teaspoon garlic powder
- 1 teaspoon ground cumin
- Salt and ground black pepper, as required
- For Sauce:
- 1/3 cup orange marmalade
- 1/3 cup honey
- 1/3 cup brown sugar

- 2 tablespoons cornstarch
- 2 tablespoons soy sauce
- 1-2 tablespoons hot sauce
- 1 tablespoon Worcestershire sauce

Directions:

1. For meatballs: in a large bowl, add all the ingredients and mix until well combined.
2. Make 1½-inch balls from the mixture.
3. Arrange half of the meatballs onto a cooking tray in a single layer.
4. Arrange the drip pan in the bottom of Instant Vortex Plus Air Fryer Oven cooking chamber.
5. Select "Air Fry" and then adjust the temperature to 380 degrees F.
6. Set the timer for 15 minutes and press the "Start".
7. When the display shows "Add Food" insert the cooking tray in the center position.
8. When the display shows "Turn Food" turn the meatballs.
9. When cooking time is complete, remove the tray from Vortex.
10. Repeat with the remaining meatballs.

11. Meanwhile, for sauce: in a small pan, add all the ingredients over medium heat and cook until thickened, stirring continuously.
12. Serve the meatballs with the topping of sauce.

Nutrition: Calories 411 Fat 11.1 g Carbs 38.8 g Protein 38.9 g

71. **Buttered Salmon**

Basic Recipe

Preparation Time: 5 minutes

Cooking Time: 10 minutes

Serving: 2

Ingredients:

- 2 salmon fillets (6-oz)
- Salt and ground black pepper, as required
- 1 tbsp butter, melted

Directions:

1. Season each salmon fillet with salt and black pepper and then, coat with the butter. Arrange the salmon fillets onto the greased cooking tray.

2. Arrange the drip pan in the bottom of the Instant Vortex Air Fryer Oven cooking chamber. Select "Air Fry" and then adjust the temperature to 360 °F. Set the time for 10 minutes and press "Start".

3. When the display shows "Add Food" insert the cooking tray in the center position. When the display shows "Turn Food" turn the salmon fillets.

4. When cooking time is complete, remove the tray from the Vortex Oven. Serve hot.

Nutrition: Calories 276 Carbs 0g Fat 16.3g Protein 33.1g

72. Lemony Salmon

Basic Recipe

Preparation Time: 5 minutes

Cooking Time: 10 minutes

Serving: 2

Ingredients:

- 1 tbsp. of fresh lemon juice
- ½ tbsp olive oil
- Salt and ground black pepper, as required
- 1 garlic clove, minced
- ½ tsp. fresh thyme leaves, chopped
- 2 (7-oz) Salmon fillets

Directions:

1. In a bowl, add all ingredients except the salmon and mix well. Add the salmon fillets and coat with the mixture generously.

2. Arrange the salmon fillets onto a lightly greased cooking rack, skin-side down. Arrange the drip pan in the bottom of the Instant Vortex Air Fryer Oven cooking chamber. Select "Air Fry" and then adjust the

temperature to 400 °F. Set the time for 10 minutes and press "Start".

3. When the display shows "Add Food" insert the cooking rack in the bottom position. When the display shows "Turn Food" turn the fillets.

4. When the cooking time is complete, remove the tray from the Vortex Oven. Serve hot.

Nutrition: Calories 297 Carbs 0.8g Fat 15.8g Protein 38.7g

73. <u>Miso Glazed Salmon</u>

Basic Recipe

Preparation Time: 5 minutes

Cooking Time: 10 minutes

Serving: 4

Ingredients:

- 1/3 cup sake
- ¼ cup sugar
- ¼ cup red miso
- 1 tbsp low-sodium soy sauce
- 2 tbsp vegetable oil
- 4 (5-oz) Skinless salmon fillets, (1-inch thick)

Directions:

1. Place the sake, sugar, miso, soy sauce and oil into a bowl and beat until thoroughly combined. Rub the salmon fillets with the mixture generously. In a plastic zip lock bag, place the salmon fillets with any remaining miso mixture.

2. Seal the bag and refrigerate to marinate for about 30 minutes Grease a baking dish that will fit in the Vortex Air Fryer Oven. Remove the salmon fillets from bag

and shake off the excess marinade. Arrange the salmon fillets into the prepared baking dish.

3. Arrange the drip pan in the bottom of the Instant Vortex Air Fryer Oven cooking chamber. Select "Broil" and Set the time for 5 minutes.

4. When the display shows "Add Food" insert the baking dish in the center position.

5. When the display shows "Turn Food" do not turn food. When cooking time is complete, remove the baking dish from the Vortex Oven. Serve hot.

Nutrition: Calories 335 Carbs 18.3g Fat 16.6g Protein 29.8g

74. Spiced Tilapia

Basic Recipe

Preparation Time: 5 minutes

Cooking Time: 12 minutes

Serving: 2

Ingredients:

- ½ Tsp lemon pepper seasoning
- ½ tsp. Garlic powder
- ½ tsp onion powder
- Salt and ground black pepper, as required
- 2 (6-oz) tilapia fillets
- 1 tbsp olive oil

Directions:

1. In a small bowl, mix together the spices, salt and black pepper. Coat the tilapia fillets with oil and then rub with spice mixture. Arrange the tilapia fillets onto a lightly greased cooking rack, skin-side down.

2. Arrange the drip pan in the bottom of the Instant Vortex Air Fryer Oven cooking chamber. Select "Air Fry" and then adjust the temperature to 360 °F. Set the time for 12 minutes and press "Start".

3. When the display shows "Add Food" insert the cooking rack in the bottom position. When the display shows "Turn Food" turn the fillets.

4. When cooking time is complete, remove the tray from the Vortex Oven. Serve hot.

Nutrition: Calories 206 Carbs 0.2g Fat 8.6g Protein 31.9g

75. Crispy Tilapia

Basic Recipe

Preparation Time: 5 minutes

Cooking Time: 15 minutes

Serving: 2

Ingredients:

- ¾ cup cornflakes, crushed
- 1 (1-oz.) packet, dry ranch-style dressing mix
- 2½ tbsp vegetable oil
- 2eggs
- 4 (6-oz) tilapia fillets

Directions:

1. In a shallow bowl, beat the eggs. In another bowl, add the cornflakes, ranch dressing, and oil and mix until a crumbly mixture form. Dip the fish fillets into egg and then, coat with the cornflake mixture.

2. Arrange the tilapia fillets onto the greased cooking tray. Arrange the drip pan in the bottom of the Instant Vortex Air Fryer Oven cooking chamber. Select "Air Fry" and then adjust the temperature to 355 °F. Set the time for 14 minutes and press "Start".

3. When the display shows "Add Food" insert the cooking tray in the center position. When the display shows "Turn Food" turn the tilapia fillets. When cooking time is complete, remove the tray from the Vortex Oven. Serve hot.

Nutrition: Calories 291 Carbs 4.9g Fat 14.6g Protein 34.8g

76. Simple Haddock

Basic Recipe

Preparation Time: 5 minutes

Cooking Time: 10 minutes

Serving: 2

Ingredients:

- 2 (6-oz) haddock fillets
- 1 tbsp olive oil
- Salt and ground black pepper, as required

Directions:

1. Coat the haddock fillets with oil and then, sprinkle with salt and black pepper. Arrange the haddock fillets onto a greased cooking rack and spray with cooking spray.

2. Arrange the drip pan in the bottom of the Instant Vortex Air Fryer Oven cooking chamber. Select "Air Fry" and then adjust the temperature to 355 °F. Set the time for 8 minutes and press "Start".

3. When the display shows "Add Food" insert the cooking rack in the center position.

4. When the display shows "Turn Food" do not turn food.

5. When the cooking time is complete, remove the rack from the Vortex Oven. Serve hot.

Nutrition: Calories 251 Carbs 0g Fat 8.6g Protein 41.2g

77. Crispy Haddock

Basic Recipe

Preparation Time: 5 minutes

Cooking Time: 10 minutes

Serving: 3

Ingredients:

- ½ Cup flour
- ½ tsp. Paprika
- 1 egg, beaten
- ¼ cup mayonnaise
- 4 oz salt and vinegar potato chips, crushed finely
- 1 lb. haddock fillet cut into 6 pieces

Direction:

1. In a shallow dish, mix together the flour and paprika. In a second shallow dish, add the egg and mayonnaise and beat well. In a third shallow dish, place the crushed potato chips.

2. Coat the fish pieces with flour mixture, then dip into egg mixture and finally coat with the potato chips. Arrange the fish pieces onto 2 cooking trays.

3. Arrange the drip pan in the bottom of the Instant Vortex Air Fryer Oven cooking chamber. Select "Air Fry" and then adjust the temperature to 370 °F. Set the time for 10 minutes and press "Start".

4. When the display shows "Add Food" insert 1 cooking tray in the top position and another in the bottom position.

5. When the display shows "Turn Food" do not turn the food but switch the position of cooking trays. When cooking time is complete, remove the trays from the Vortex Oven. Serve hot.

Nutrition: Calories 456 Carbs 40.9g Fat 22.7g Protein 43.5g

78. <u>Vinegar Halibut</u>

Basic Recipe

Preparation Time: 5 minutes

Cooking Time: 12 minutes

Serving: 2

Ingredients:

- 2 (5-oz) Halibut fillets
- 1 garlic clove, minced
- 1 tsp fresh rosemary, minced
- 1 tbsp olive oil
- 1 tbsp red wine vinegar
- 1/8 tsp hot sauce

Directions:

1. In a large resealable bag, add all ingredients. Seal the bag and shale well to mix. Refrigerate to marinate for at least 30 minutes Remove the fish fillets from the bag and shake off the excess marinade. Arrange the halibut fillets onto the greased cooking tray.

2. Arrange the drip pan in the bottom of the Instant Vortex Air Fryer Oven cooking chamber. Select "Bake" and then adjust the temperature to 450 °F. Set

the time for 12 minutes and press "Start". When the display shows "Add Food" insert the cooking tray in the center position. When the display shows "Turn Food" turn the halibut fillets. When the cooking time is complete, remove the tray from the Vortex Oven. Serve hot.

Nutrition: Calories 223 Carbs 1g Fat 10.4g Protein 30g

79. <u>Breaded Cod</u>

Basic Recipe

Preparation Time: 5 minutes

Cooking Time: 10 minutes

Serving: 4

Ingredients:

- 1/3 cup all-purpose flour
- Ground black pepper, as required
- 1 large egg
- 2 tbsp water
- 2/3 cup cornflakes, crushed
- 1 tbsp parmesan cheese, grated
- 1/8 tsp cayenne pepper
- 1 lb. Cod fillets –
- Salt, as required

Directions:

1. In a shallow dish, add the flour and black pepper and mix well. In a second shallow dish, add the egg and water and beat well. In a third shallow dish, add the cornflakes, cheese and cayenne pepper and mix well.

2. Season the cod fillets with salt evenly. Coat the fillets with flour mixture, then dip into egg mixture and finally coat with the cornflake mixture.

3. Arrange the cod fillets onto the greased cooking rack. Arrange the drip pan in the bottom of the Instant Vortex Air Fryer Oven cooking chamber. Select "Air Fry" and then adjust the temperature to 400 °F. Set the time for 10 minutes and press "Start".

4. When the display shows "Add Food" insert the cooking rack in the bottom position. When the display shows "Turn Food" turn the cod fillets. When cooking time is complete, remove the tray from the Vortex Oven. Serve hot.

Nutrition: Calories 168 Carbs 12.1g Fat 2.7g Protein 23.7g

80. Spicy Catfish

Basic Recipe

Preparation Time: 5 minutes

Cooking Time: 15 minutes

Serving: 4

Ingredients:

- 2 tbsp cornmeal polenta
- 2 tsp Cajun seasoning
- ½ tsp paprika
- ½ tsp garlic powder
- Salt, as required
- 2 (6-oz) catfish fillets
- 1 tbsp olive oil

Directions:

1. In a bowl, mix together the cornmeal, Cajun seasoning, paprika, garlic powder, and salt. Add the catfish fillets and coat evenly with the mixture. Now, coat each fillet with oil.

2. Arrange the fish fillets onto a greased cooking rack and spray with cooking spray. Arrange the drip pan in the bottom of the Instant Vortex Air Fryer Oven cooking

chamber. Select "Air Fry" and then adjust the temperature to 400 °F. Set the timer for 14 minutes and press "Start".

3. When the display shows "Add Food" insert the cooking rack in the center position. When the display shows "Turn Food" turn the fillets.

4. When cooking time is complete, remove the rack from the Vortex Oven. Serve hot.

Nutrition: Calories 32 Carbs 6.7g Fat 20.3g Protein 27.3g

81. Delicious Fajita Chicken

Preparation Time: 10 minutes

Cooking Time: 15 minutes

Servings: 4

Ingredients:

- 4 chicken breasts, boneless & sliced
- 1 bell pepper, sliced
- 2 tbsp fajita seasoning
- 2 tbsp olive oil
- 1 onion, sliced

Directions:

1. Line multi-level air fryer basket with parchment paper.
2. In a bowl, add chicken and remaining ingredients and toss well.
3. Add chicken mixture into the basket.
4. Place basket into the pot. Secure pot with air fryer lid and cook on air fry mode at 380 F for 15 minutes. Flip halfway through.
5. Serve and enjoy.

Nutrition: Calories 374 Fat 17.9 g Carbohydrates 8 g Sugar 2.7 g Protein 42.8 g Cholesterol 130 mg

82. Chinese Chicken Wings

Preparation Time: 10 minutes

Cooking Time: 30 minutes

Servings: 2

Ingredients:

- 4 chicken wings
- 1 tbsp soy sauce
- 1 tbsp Chinese spice
- 1 tsp mixed spice
- Pepper
- Salt

Directions:

1. Line multi-level air fryer basket with parchment paper.
2. Add chicken wings and remaining ingredients into the mixing bowl and toss well.
3. Transfer chicken wings into the basket.
4. Place basket into the pot. Secure pot with air fryer lid and cook on air fry mode at 350 F for 30 minutes. Flip halfway through.
5. Serve and enjoy.

Nutrition: Calories 567 Fat 22.1 g Carbohydrates 0.9 g Sugar 0.2 g Protein 85.7 g Cholesterol 260 mg

83. Caribbean Chicken Thighs

Preparation Time: 10 minutes

Cooking Time: 10 minutes

Servings: 8

Ingredients:

- 3 lbs. chicken thigh, skinless and boneless
- 1 tbsp cayenne
- 1 tbsp cinnamon
- 1 tbsp coriander powder
- 3 tbsp coconut oil, melted
- 1/2 tsp ground nutmeg
- 1/2 tsp ground ginger
- Pepper
- Salt

Directions:

1. Line multi-level air fryer basket with parchment paper.
2. In a small bowl, mix together all ingredients except chicken.
3. Rub bowl mixture all over the chicken thighs.
4. Add chicken thighs into the basket.

5. Place basket into the pot. Secure pot with air fryer lid and cook on air fry mode at 390 F for 10 minutes. Flip halfway through.

6. Serve and enjoy.

Nutrition: Calories 373 Fat 17.9 g Carbohydrates 1.2 g Sugar 0.1 g Protein 49.3 g Cholesterol 151 mg

84. Garlic Herb Chicken Breasts

Preparation Time: 10 minutes

Cooking Time: 15 minutes

Servings: 6

Ingredients:

- 2 lbs. chicken breasts, skinless and boneless
- 3 garlic cloves, minced
- 1/4 cup yogurt
- 2 tsp garlic herb seasoning
- 1 tsp onion powder
- 1/4 cup mayonnaise
- 1/4 tsp salt

Directions:

1. Line multi-level air fryer basket with parchment paper.
2. In a small bowl, mix mayonnaise, seasoning, onion powder, garlic, and yogurt.
3. Brush chicken with mayonnaise mixture and season with salt.
4. Place chicken breasts into the basket.

5. Place basket into the pot. Secure pot with air fryer lid and cook on air fry mode at 380 F for 15 minutes. Flip halfway through.

6. Serve and enjoy.

Nutrition: Calories 336 Fat 14.6 g Carbohydrates 3.9 g Sugar 1.5 g Protein 44.6 g Cholesterol 138 mg

85. Crispy Chicken Tenders

Preparation Time: 10 minutes

Cooking Time: 15 minutes

Servings: 6

Ingredients:

- 8 oz chicken breast tenderloins
- 1 egg, lightly beaten
- 1 cup almond flour
- 1/4 cup heavy whipping cream
- 1 tsp pepper
- 1 tsp salt

Directions:

1. Line multi-level air fryer basket with parchment paper.
2. In a bowl, whisk egg, heavy whipping cream, pepper, and salt.
3. In a shallow dish, add the almond flour.
4. Dip chicken in egg mixture then coats with almond flour mixture.
5. Place coated chicken into the basket.

6. Place basket into the pot. Secure pot with air fryer lid and cook on air fry mode at 400 F for 15 minutes. Flip halfway through.

7. Serve and enjoy.

Nutrition: Calories 89 Fat 5.1 g Carbohydrates 1.4 g Sugar 0.2 g Protein 9.5 g Cholesterol 58 mg

86. Cheese Herb Chicken Wings

Preparation Time: 10 minutes

Cooking Time: 15 minutes

Servings: 4

Ingredients:

- 2 lbs. chicken wings
- 1/2 cup parmesan cheese, grated
- 1 tsp herb de Provence
- 1 tsp smoked paprika
- Salt

Directions:

1. Line multi-level air fryer basket with parchment paper.
2. In a small bowl, mix cheese, herb de Provence, paprika, and salt.
3. Coat chicken wings with cheese mixture and place it into the basket.
4. Place basket into the pot. Secure pot with air fryer lid and cook on air fry mode at 350 F for 15 minutes. Flip halfway through.
5. Serve and enjoy.

Nutrition: Calories 472 Fat 19.5 g Carbohydrates 0.7 g Sugar 0.1 g Protein 69.7 g Cholesterol 210 mg

87. Delicious Mustard Chicken Tenders

Preparation Time: 10 minutes

Cooking Time: 20 minutes

Servings: 4

Ingredients:

- 1 lbs. chicken tenders
- 1/2 tsp paprika
- 1 garlic clove, minced
- 2 tbsp fresh tarragon, chopped
- 1/2 cup whole grain mustard
- 1/2 oz fresh lemon juice
- 1/2 tsp pepper
- 1/4 tsp kosher salt

Directions:

1. Line multi-level air fryer basket with parchment paper.
2. Add all ingredients except chicken to the large bowl and mix well.
3. Add chicken to the bowl and stir until well coated.
4. Place coated chicken tenders into the multi-level air fryer basket.

5. Place basket into the pot. Secure pot with air fryer lid and cook on bake mode at 400 F for 15-20 minutes.

6. Serve and enjoy.

Nutrition: Calories 242 Fat 9.5 g Carbohydrates 3.1 g Sugar 0.1 g Protein 33.2 g Cholesterol 101 mg

88. Baked Chicken Tenders

Preparation Time: 10 minutes

Cooking Time: 35 minutes

Servings: 4

Ingredients:

- 2 lbs. chicken tenders
- 2 tbsp olive oil
- 3 dill sprigs
- 1 large zucchini
- 1 cup grape tomatoes
- For topping:
- 1 tbsp fresh lemon juice
- 1 tbsp fresh dill, chopped
- 2 tbsp feta cheese, crumbled
- 1 tbsp olive oil

Directions:

1. Line multi-level air fryer basket with parchment paper.

2. Coat chicken with oil and season with salt and place into the multi-level air fryer basket. Add zucchini, dill, and tomatoes on top of chicken.

3. Place basket into the pot. Secure pot with air fryer lid and cook on bake mode at 400 F for 30 minutes.

4. Meanwhile, in a small bowl, stir together all topping ingredients.

5. Place chicken onto the serving plate then top with vegetables and discard dill sprigs.

6. Sprinkle topping mixture on top of chicken and vegetables.

7. Serve and enjoy.

Nutrition: Calories 563 Fat 28.7 g Carbohydrates 6.5 g Sugar 2.9 g Protein 68.3 g Cholesterol 206 mg

89. <u>Paprika Chicken Breasts</u>

Preparation Time: 10 minutes

Cooking Time: 35 minutes

Servings: 4

Ingredients:

- 4 chicken breasts, skinless and boneless, cut into chunks
- 2 tbsp smoked paprika
- 3 tbsp olive oil
- 2 tsp garlic, minced
- 2 tbsp lemon juice
- Pepper
- Salt

Directions:

1. Line multi-level air fryer basket with parchment paper.
2. In a small bowl, mix garlic, paprika, lemon juice, and olive oil.
3. Season chicken with pepper and salt and rub with garlic mixture.
4. Place chicken breasts into the multi-level air fryer basket.

5. Place basket into the pot. Secure pot with air fryer lid and cook on bake mode at 350 F for 30-35 minutes.

6. Serve and enjoy.

Nutrition: Calories 381 Fat 21.8 g Carbohydrates 2.6 g Sugar 0.5 g Protein 42.9 g Cholesterol 130 mg

90. Lemon Garlic Chicken Drumsticks

Preparation Time: 10 minutes

Cooking Time: 40 minutes

Servings: 4

Ingredients:

- 2 lbs. chicken drumsticks
- 10 garlic cloves, sliced
- 2 tbsp olive oil
- 1 fresh lemon juice
- 2 tbsp parsley, chopped

Directions:

1. Line multi-level air fryer basket with parchment paper.
2. Place chicken in the multi-level air fryer basket.
3. Sprinkle parsley and garlic over the chicken.
4. Pour lemon juice and olive oil on top of chicken.
5. Place basket into the pot. Secure pot with air fryer lid and cook on bake mode at 400 F for 35-40 minutes.
6. Serve and enjoy.

Nutrition: Calories 458 Fat 20.1 g Carbohydrates 2.9 g Sugar 0.4 g Protein 63 g Cholesterol 200 mg

91. Perfect Salmon Dinner

Preparation time: 10 minutes

Cooking time: 2 minutes

Servings: 3

Ingredients:

- 1 lb. salmon fillet, cut into three pieces
- 2 garlic cloves, minced
- 1/2 tsp ground cumin
- 1 tsp red chili powder
- Pepper
- Salt

Directions:

1. Pour 1 1/2 cups water into the instant pot then place trivet into the pot.
2. In a small bowl, mix together garlic, cumin, chili powder, pepper, and salt.
3. Rub salmon with spice mixture and place on top of the trivet.

4. Seal pot with lid and cook on steam mode for 2 minutes.

5. Once done then release pressure using the quick-release method than open the lid.

6. Serve and enjoy.

Nutrition: Calories 207 Fat 9.6 g Carbohydrates 1.3 g Sugar 0.1 g Protein 29.6 g Cholesterol 67 mg

92. <u>Steam Clams</u>

Preparation time: 10 minutes

Cooking time: 3 minutes

Servings: 3

Ingredients:

- 1 lb. mushy shell clams
- 2 tbsp butter, melted
- 1/4 cup white wine
- 1/2 tsp garlic powder
- 1/4 cup fresh lemon juice

Directions:

1. Add white wine, lemon juice, garlic powder, and butter into the instant pot.
2. Place trivet into the pot.
3. Arrange clams on top of the trivet.
4. Seal pot with lid and cook on manual high pressure for 3 minutes.
5. Once done then allow to release pressure naturally then open the lid.
6. Serve and enjoy.

Nutrition: Calories 336 Fat 18.5 g Carbohydrates 24.8 g Sugar 2.8 g Protein 13.1 g Cholesterol 20 mg

93. Delicious Tilapia

Preparation Time: 10 minutes

Cooking Time: 8 minutes

Serving: 4

Ingredients:

- 2 tilapia fillets
- 1/4 tsp cayenne
- 1/2 tsp cumin
- 1 tsp garlic powder
- 1 tsp dried oregano
- 2 tsp brown sugar
- 2 tbsp paprika
- Salt

Directions:

1. In a small bowl, mix together cayenne, cumin, garlic powder, oregano, sugar, paprika, and salt and rub over tilapia fillets.
2. Place the dehydrating tray in a multi-level air fryer basket and place basket in the instant pot.
3. Place tilapia fillets on dehydrating tray.

4. Seal pot with air fryer lid and select air fry mode then set the temperature to 400 F and timer for 8 minutes. Turn tilapia fillets halfway through.

5. Serve and enjoy.

Nutrition: Calories 67 Fat 1.1 g Carbohydrates 4.3 g Sugar 2 g Protein 11.2 g Cholesterol 28 mg

94. <u>Horseradish Salmon</u>

Preparation Time: 10 minutes

Cooking Time: 7 minutes

Serving: 2

Ingredients:

- 2 salmon fillets
- 1/4 cup breadcrumbs
- 2 tbsp olive oil
- 1 tbsp horseradish
- Pepper
- Salt

Directions:

1. Place the dehydrating tray in a multi-level air fryer basket and place basket in the instant pot.
2. Place salmon fillets on dehydrating tray.
3. In a small bowl, mix together breadcrumbs, oil, horseradish, pepper, and salt and spread over salmon fillets.
4. Seal pot with air fryer lid and select air fry mode then set the temperature to 400 F and timer for 7 minutes.
5. Serve and enjoy.

Nutrition: Calories 413 Fat 25.8 g Carbohydrates 10.6 g Sugar 1.4 g Protein 36.4 g Cholesterol 78 mg

95. Shrimp Scampi

Preparation time: 10 minutes

Cooking time: 2 minutes

Servings: 2

Ingredients:

- 1 lb. shrimp, peeled and deveined
- 1 cup of water
- 1/4 tsp red chili flakes
- 3 garlic cloves, minced
- 2 tbsp butter
- 2 tbsp lemon juice
- Pepper
- Salt

Directions:

1. Add butter into the instant pot and set the pot on sauté mode.
2. Add garlic, pepper, red chili flakes, and salt to the pot and sauté for 2 minutes.
3. Add shrimp and water. Stir well.
4. Seal pot with lid and cook on manual high pressure for 2 minutes.

5. Once done then release pressure using the quick-release method than open the lid.

6. Stir in lemon juice and serve.

Nutrition: Calories 382 Fat 15.5 g Carbohydrates 5.3 g Sugar 0.4 g Protein 52.2 g Cholesterol 508 mg

96. Dijon Fish Fillets

Preparation time: 10 minutes

Cooking time: 3 minutes

Servings: 2

Ingredients:

- 2 halibut fillets
- 1 tbsp Dijon mustard
- 1 1/2 cups water
- Pepper
- Salt

Directions:

1. Pour water into the instant pot then place steamer basket in the pot.
2. Season fish fillets with pepper and salt and brush with Dijon mustard.
3. Place fish fillets in the steamer basket.
4. Seal pot with lid and cook on manual high pressure for 3 minutes.
5. Once done then release pressure using the quick-release method than open the lid.
6. Serve and enjoy.

Nutrition: Calories 323 Fat 7 g Carbohydrates 0.5 g Sugar 0.1 g Protein 60.9 g Cholesterol 93 mg

97. Garlic Parmesan Shrimp

Preparation time: 10 minutes

Cooking time: 10 minutes

Servings: 4

Ingredients:

- 1lb shrimp, deveined and peeled
- 1 tablespoon olive oil
- 1 teaspoon salt
- 1 teaspoon fresh cracked pepper
- 1 tablespoon lemon juice
- 6 cloves garlic, diced
- 1/2 cup grated parmesan cheese
- 1/4 cup diced cilantro

Directions:

1. Toss the shrimp with oil and all other ingredients in a bowl.
2. Spread the seasoned shrimp in the air fryer basket.
3. Press "power button" of air fry oven and turn the dial to select the "air roast" mode.
4. Press the time button and again turn the dial to set the cooking time to 10 minutes.

5. Now push the temp button and rotate the dial to set the temperature at 350 degrees f.

6. Once preheated, place the air fryer basket in the oven and close its lid.

7. Toss and flip the shrimp when cooked halfway through.

8. Serve warm.

Nutrition: Calories 184 Total fat 6.2g Saturated fat 1.6g Cholesterol 241mg Sodium 893mg Total carbohydrate 3.5g Dietary fiber 0.1g Total sugars 0.1g Protein 27.3g

98. Bang Bang Breaded Shrimp

Preparation time: 10 minutes

Cooking time: 14 minutes

Servings: 4

Ingredients:

- 1 lb. Raw shrimp peeled and deveined
- 1 egg white
- 1/2 cup flour
- 3/4 cup panko bread crumbs
- 1 teaspoon paprika
- Montreal seasoning to taste
- Salt and pepper to taste
- Cooking spray
- Bang bang sauce
- 1/3 cup Greek yogurt
- 2 tablespoon sriracha
- 1/4 cup sweet chili sauce

Directions:

1. Mix flour with salt, black pepper, paprika, and Montreal seasoning in a bowl.
2. Dredge the shrimp the flour then dips in the egg.

3. Coat the shrimp with the breadcrumbs and place them in an air fryer basket.
4. Press "power button" of air fry oven and turn the dial to select the "air roast" mode.
5. Press the time button and again turn the dial to set the cooking time to 14 minutes.
6. Now push the temp button and rotate the dial to set the temperature at 400 degrees f.
7. Once preheated, place the air fryer basket in the oven and close its lid.
8. Toss and flip the shrimp when cooked halfway through.
9. Serve warm.

Nutrition: Calories 200 Total fat 2.7g Saturated fat 0.5g Cholesterol 100mg Sodium 663mg Total carbohydrate 25.1g Dietary fiber 1g Total sugars 6.1g Protein 17.4g

99. Taco Fried Shrimp

Preparation time: 10 minutes

Cooking time: 5 minutes

Servings: 6

Ingredients:

- 17 shrimp, defrosted, peeled, and deveined
- 1 cup breadcrumbs Italian
- 1 tablespoon taco seasoning
- 1 tablespoon garlic salt
- 4 tablespoon butter melted
- Olive oil spray

Directions:

1. Toss the shrimp with oil and all other ingredients in a bowl.
2. Spread the seasoned shrimp in the air fryer basket.
3. Press "power button" of air fry oven and turn the dial to select the "air roast" mode.
4. Press the time button and again turn the dial to set the cooking time to 5 minutes.
5. Now push the temp button and rotate the dial to set the temperature at 400 degrees f.

6. Once preheated, place the air fryer basket in the oven and close its lid.

7. Toss and flip the shrimp when cooked halfway through.

8. Serve warm.

Nutrition: Calories 350 Total fat 17.6g Saturated fat 10.1g Cholesterol 235mg Sodium 760mg Total carbohydrate 21.4g Dietary fiber 1g Total sugars 2g Protein 25.4g

100. Asparagus Shrimp Risotto

Preparation time: 10 minutes

Cooking time: 16 minutes

Servings: 6

Ingredients:

- 1 1/2 cups arborio rice
- 1 tbsp butter
- 3 1/2 cups chicken stock
- 1/2 cup white wine
- 1 cup mushrooms, sliced
- 1/4 cup parmesan cheese, grated
- 1 lb. shrimp, cooked
- 1 cup asparagus, chopped
- 1/2 onion, diced
- 2 tsp olive oil
- 1/2 tsp pepper
- Salt

Directions:

1. Add oil into the instant pot and set the pot on sauté mode.
2. Add onion to the pot and sauté for 2-3 minutes.

3. Add mushrooms and cook for 5 minutes.

4. Add rice and cook until lightly brown.

5. Add stock and wine and stir well.

6. Seal pot with lid and cook on manual high pressure for 6 minutes,

7. Once done then release pressure using the quick-release method than open the lid.

8. Add asparagus and butter and cook on sauté mode for 1 minute.

9. Add shrimp and cook for 1 minute.

10. Stir in cheese and serve.

Nutrition: Calories 339 Fat 6.4 g Carbohydrates 42.3 g Sugar 1.6 g Protein 23.3 g Cholesterol 168 mg

CONCLUSION

In this cookbook, we introduced a new member of the Instant Pot family, the Instant Pot Pro Crisp Air Fryer. It uses two different cooking techniques, one for pressure cooking and the other for air frying. The instant pot pro crisp air fryer comes with two lids, one for pressure cooking and another for air frying. It is one of the advanced cooking appliances that comes with 11 cooking functions.

The cookbook contains healthy, delicious and mouth-watering recipes. The book contains all types of recipes starting from breakfast to desserts. The recipes in this cookbook are unique and written with step-by-step instructions. All the recipes are described with their perfect preparation and cooking time. Each recipe ends with their exact nutritional information.

CPSIA information can be obtained
at www.ICGtesting.com
Printed in the USA
BVHW090057180621
609824BV00004B/1221